Chemical-Free Skin Health®

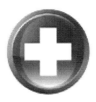

Chemical-Free Skin Health®

Stop • Challenge • Choose

by

Bob Root

Foreword by

Kathleen Beaton

M42 Publishing

Annapolis, MD

Chemical-Free Skin Health®

Stop• Challenge • Choose

M42 Publishing

an imprint of M42 Publishing

For information address:

M42 Publishing

626C Admiral Drive

Suite 315

Annapolis, MD 21401

www.M42publishing.com

info@M42publishing.com

ISBN: 978-0-9829510-0-2

Library of Congress PCN

2010912371

Dedication:

To my wife Wendy, whose courage to beat Cancer remains an inspiration to me every day. And to her wanting to stay married to "One of the crazy ones!" To Burt Rutan and Sir Richard Branson for inspiring me to look for what's right and not what's wrong. True explorers! To Dr Mauro Ferrari for teaching me about the world of potential in nano-pharmacology. To all of the scientists at Los Alamos National Labs for your skip generations thinking. To Kathleen Beaton for your guidance and intense wisdom about what goes on and in our bodies. To Brian Blanchard for your inspiring British humor. To Teunis Tel, my big Dutch friend! Perhaps the finest industrial design mind in the universe. To Ullrich Metzler for believing in the simple dream. To Marilyn Speir for your help and belief in me. To my friends and fellow companies at Safe Cosmetics for "keep on keepin on!" To the many authors contributing freely to Wikipedia for your help in simplifying the book for its intended readers.

Special Dedication:

To all my scientific, medical and aboriginal healer friends who guide me to help others and whose currency is knowledge that they share freely.

To Gordon Volkers, without your dedication and help to Keys, we would have not made it.

To Diz, You were always supervising. I will miss you for all of time!

"Chemical-Free is an industry jargon term that has many meanings to different people. To me it simply means to avoid anything that can harm you, shorten your life or shorten your youth!"

Bob Root

Chief Technology Officer

Keys Care

Disclaimer

This publication contains the opinion and ideas of its author. It is intended to provide helpful and informative material on the subjects addresses in the publication. It is sold with the understanding that the author and publisher are not engaged in rendering medical, health or any kind of personal professional services in this book. The reader should consult with his or her medical, health or other competent professional before adopting any suggestions in this book or drawing reference from it.

The author and publisher specifically disclaim all responsibility for any liability, loss, or risk, personal or otherwise, which is incurred as a consequence, directly or indirectly, of the use and application of any contents of this book.

Foreword

Foreword

by

Kathleen Beaton

(Professional makeup artist who lives and works near Los Angeles, California)

Many years ago, in the scientific community, there was a falsely held belief that the skin acted as a barrier, protecting us internally from whatever we applied to it.

If you were raised in an east coast Italian family in the late 60's and had a cold, the older generation of grandparents and great aunts and uncles, frequently mashed up garlic, put it on the bottoms of your feet and then put a pair of socks on you, as a cure all. Trust me when I tell you that within a short time, man, you could taste that garlic. The skin absorbs what we put on it. It goes into our bloodstreams. If you don't want to try the garlic test, just think about nicotine patches and birth control patches.

If only I had known those scientists back then, I could have gotten in their faces with my stinky little kid garlic breath and proven to them that they were wrong.

Every day before we even leave the house, many of us unconsciously expose ourselves to hundreds of chemicals from personal care products alone. This book will educate and empower you to take charge of your own health and the health of your loved ones. Please don't rely on the government for your personal safety. It is our individual responsibility. The FDA does not regulate the chemicals used in personal care products. Bottom line. We can change this; but for now, it is on us. Together we can create a change for future generations.

I've been working in the world of hair and makeup for over 25 years now. I do my best to honor this human design and I marvel at the body's ability to heal and constantly regenerate. So naturally, I began looking into what I was using topically.

As a professional makeup artist, I was first introduced to Bob Root and Wendy Steele's Keys brand Eye Butter at a Campaign for Safe Cosmetics meeting. I thought I'd be the only person there armed with my notepad and pen, but to my surprise, the place was packed. I wasn't the only makeup artist concerned.

I later was personally introduced to Bob and Wendy by our dear mutual friend Ele Keats.

Like Bob, as I began educating myself and reading ingredient declarations, I became fascinated with how companies got away with including known carcinogens in their formulations. I became an ingredient nerd. I bought books and researched words that I couldn't even pronounce and was pretty shocked each time I read the ingredient's function alongside the possible health concern.

When I finally sat down with Bob and Wendy we realized our passion for bringing about a change. We share a love of people, animals, the planet, delicious food, an endless desire to learn, and of course a good sense of humor to keep it all in perspective.

I am honored to call them my friends.

Keys Soap was born out of necessity for Wendy's extremely sensitive skin. Bob went back to basics and formulated clean products that nourish and heal the skin.

Bob's philosophy is that there are two components to skin health and wellness. It is a combination of what you use and what you avoid.

I invite you to read on and learn how to do just that.

It is my great pleasure to introduce you to Bob's work and begin the process of reclaiming your health.

This book is full of critical information and will empower you to make better choices. Bob presents you, the reader with data that he has acquired over his years of studying the effects chemicals in skincare have on your well-being. His is a "less is more" philosophy and I agree completely. Simplify. And after you lighten your toxic load, have a look at Keys products. They are amazing.

To your health, or as my Italian relatives with garlic on the soles of their feet would say,

"A Votre Sante."

Preface

"I have come to the belief that many skin disorders are misdiagnosed and probably caused by chemicals in cosmetics, personal care, household products and chemicals in our environment."

Bob Root

Purpose:

The purpose of this book is to share freely my perceptions of the chemicals that our skin is exposed to every day without our knowledge or choice. I have intended to simplify industry jargon and terms to keep everything in perspective. The purpose of this book is also to elevate the base knowledge level of people new to the concept that everything we put on our bodies has the same impact as what we put in it. I also hope to alter the belief that more cosmetics make us younger looking to just maybe believe that the opposite is closer to the truth.

Thoughts:

I have written this book without the assistance of professional editors and writers. Although with my Hollywood connections I have a wide range of pros to choose from, the thread of this book is really a story of my discovery in joining the cosmetics industry and what I learned along the way. These are my discoveries, my observations and my impressions. Having some of these altered by another concerned me. So, I thought to just write it.

As you read this book, keep in mind my two favorite quotes of all time:

"For some years now, I have been afflicted with the belief that flight is possible to man."

Wilbur Wright

"The sign of an uncreative mind is a man that cannot figure out how to spell a word more than one way."

Mark Twain

Lastly, I attempted to do something in this book that a friend told me is impossible. That is to write a thread of a story and to let each chapter be able to stand on its own. So feel free to jump to the chapters that interest you or read it as you please. The book and my message should hold together no matter your reading style.

I use the word truth and Truth (capital T) in this book as little as possible. It does sneak in here and there. As a theoretical scientist, there is not absolute truth. Only what we now know to be true and that will undoubtedly be disproven by some graduate student somewhere in the ether. Said, I am a firm believer that perception is reality.

Acknowledgements

To all of the companies and people who support and grow The Compact for Safe Cosmetics. To the Environmental Working Group for providing a database for safe cosmetics and personal care that provides people and the industry with information to help make the best choices. To all my friends that range from naturopaths, to herbalist, to doctors, to scientists and those that explore the quantum world. Lastly, to all the crazy ones that ask the question "Why Not?" instead of why.

Introduction

Chemical-Free Skin Health®: Snapshot

Our skin is our largest and most vulnerable organ. Love it and it will love you. Protect it and it will protect you. Abuse it and it will shorten your life.

There have been more chemicals developed in the last twenty years than in all of mankind. Of the 20,000 chemicals in use in the cosmetic, personal care and household products industry, less than 1% have been tested for safety. A few years ago, I read something from the Center for Disease Control that ~63% of Americans claim to have a skin disorder. A Connection? Probably!

There are no US Government regulations for skin care or household products.

What I have come to believe is that more than 50% of skin disorders are misdiagnosed and are caused by chemicals in the products we use every day.

An unlikely title? Not really! When you read this book, the title will become very appropriate and clear to you. It is clearly possible to reduce the chemical body burden, but it takes work.

This book is a perspective on the chemical world we live in and why I believe all of us should be concerned for our lives and the lives of our families, friends and the animals that share our lives. This book is not intended to scare you, although it might. It is really to draw attention to what our lives have become and the chemicals, companies and products that rule it.

It is about having a choice and making choices that improve our lives.

When I started this book, I felt totally unqualified to write it. After all, I am not a chemist nor do I fully understand the art and science of chemistry. I do understand, study and live in the quantum world of small particles, machines and reactions. I think this gives me a perspective that might just be new and unique. As I climb to 100,000 feet and look back at the history of chemicals in our lives, I realize how relatively short lived this industry has been operating under the new chemical standards. It is merely a blip in history.

Even in its short life, concerned people have periodically raised questions about chemicals that are supposed to be safe that turned out to harm us and even harm generations. Whether it was a pesticide like DDT or a prescription drug called Thalidomide, these chemicals were later found to cause severe harm to humans in one form or the other.

 It is also not just about what is wrong. I am reminded of outliers like Adelle Davis. Adelle Davis was the author of four bestselling books: "Let's Cook It Right", "Let's Have Healthy Children", "Let's Get Well", and "Let's Eat Right To Keep Fit".

Adelle Davis was a visionary born in 1904. When going back through her history it is amazing to realize the impact Adelle had on the most recent and popular diets that are the craze now. Adelle Davis was the pioneer of the nutritional revolution. Her teachings and writings influenced people striving for health and wellness long before my time. The point? We have to look at what we put on our skin both good and bad. Eliminate some things and add others changing our behavior.

As I began to write, I began to feel a bit more like a reporter. This then changed quickly to a responsibility to shine a spotlight on what I was seeing as a non-chemist formulator of natural skin care and pet care products. I felt as if there was no thread or conclusion that I could draw from the book until I had finished it. This is when the purpose of this book became clear to me.

Simply put, whether you read past this introduction or not, the one thing that you should glean from it is that we as individuals are responsible for our own lives. This includes what we put on to and in our bodies or what we choose to be exposed to in the environments in which we live. Take charge of your life is the message. If you choose to trust that the government will protect you, that a doctor will cure you or one of those activists will shed light on what is wrong in our world, you are naive at best.

Sorry if I shock you. I merely want to open all of our eyes that there is no free lunch, nothing that is harmless and that one creature poison is another medicine. It is finding out what is right for you in your life. Today there is no excuse with more and more knowledge at our fingertips.

Every day through the eyes of my customers, I meet people that have had a life-threatening event that wakes them up to take charge of their lives. Story after story of wins and losses of life bring tears of pain and tears of joy. Therefore, I hope this book will help to open your eyes to take charge of what you are exposed to everyday. I ask you to Stop, Challenge and Choose everything that you hear when it comes to products that you put in and on your body. There is no singular Truth only what is true today. Tomorrow will be different. For that, I am sure.

I have been in the personal care industry for only six years, but as a student of science, I offer my opinion of what I see. These forces of good and bad are truly the basis of a chemical war.

It is about choices!

Chapter 1: The Big "C"! How I Became Unlikely Formulator

Defining Moments is a book I co-authored with my wife, Wendy, in 1999. It is a story about a chance meeting in Santa Fe New Mexico and a 3000-mile romance that culminated in us leaving our high-powered corporate careers to live on a boat in San Diego. Both living an "Up in the Air" lifestyle, my high tech Silicon Valley CEO position and Wendy's VP of Coca-Cola role were of little consequence compared to the news of the Big C...Cancer!

Living an idyllic lifestyle on a motor yacht on San Diego's Harbor Island, one day I noticed a waxy mark near Wendy's left ankle. Calling her attention to it, I held a mirror next to this thin strange spot that was about the size of a pencil eraser. Within a week it was bright red. Another week passed as she was at Scripps Clinic being examined by Dr. Hugh Greenway. This renowned dermatologist and Mohs surgeon trained directly by Fred Mohs delivered the diagnosis. It was Melanoma at the very earliest stage. Another week and she was back on the boat, leg elevated and the Cancer gone.

What happened then was another defining moment for us. Little did I know that I would be developing, designing and manufacturing skin care products that would make people feel good and solve many of their skin problems. Little did I know that I would be writing a book about natural skincare. After all, I am an unlikely candidate.

Wendy's diagnosis, surgery and treatment were somewhat a success. I say somewhat because, yes the Melanoma was gone, but the reaction that she had to the prescription and over-the-counter products left her in tears, aging before her time and with so many diagnosed new skin disorders that we were spending nearly $1,000.00 a month on products meant to reverse all of these problems.

Was it the Cancer or the products? 100% the products! Why? The chemicals in them! Many of the active ingredients had side effects, but what we learned later is that it was the ingredients making up the lotions, formulas and skincare products that were causing most of her physical and mental distress.

Disease to us started with Cancer and soon became two words. Dis Ease!

After three years of doctors, skincare specialists, estheticians, herbalists, naturopaths and witchdoctors, I stepped in. Wendy's skin was now paper thin. She had adult acne, psoriasis, eczema, dermatitis and reacted to a slight scratching on her neck and arms as if she had been mauled by a cougar. An itch was always followed by huge raised welts.

In Silicon Valley, we would joke that engineers subtract! What this means is that when a new project would begin, we would start with a clean slate and not add to an existing product. From the earth up was a practice and credo. So, that training and discipline came into play one day when Wendy returned from Johns Hopkins with another bag full of prescriptions and products all with warnings that should scare the hell out of even the numbest of us. I looked at her and said one word that would forever change both of our lives. One word that started her recovery. One word that inspired our products. One word that began our company. One word that thrust us into the center of a new industry and one word that was the beginning of this book.

The word? STOP! Stop everything! I said, put all that shit they have been giving you in a box now! We are going back to the basics. We are going to watch everything you put in and on your body like a hawk. I want to know what is in everything and if it is not listed on the label, you are not going to use it. It is not my nature to demand and yet Wendy listened, studied, learned and quickly became an expert at what was good for her and what was not. More important, she learned why.

Natural products were not our quest. In fact, we quickly realized that the terms natural and organic were neither a feature nor a benefit. We found that many products claiming to be natural were not. We found that they contained most of the ingredients in the prescription products or worse, the lack of ingredients exposed her to microbiology exposure like staph and E.coli. The answers were and are not black and white. What was clear to both of us is that the deeper we dug into products, regimes and the industry that no one had the answers.

I set out to develop products that would work for Wendy. Not a chemist, I took a Silicon Valley engineering approach to a solution. Starting with Dr Bronner's soap, Wendy stopped using every product and hid them from herself. Out of sight, out of mind! Bronner's helped! It really did. The results were remarkable. Then it seemed to be a miracle and now I know why. Initially, Wendy reacted a bit to the soap. Thinking that it was her super sensitive skin, we later realized that her skin was so damaged by the prescription products that Bronner's soap turned out to be a little too aggressive and alkaline for her. So, I looked to the origins of Dr Bronner's Castile type soap and traced them back nearly 400 years. Starting with that old Spanish Castile recipe, I began to formulate around this ancient remedy using modern technology and pharmaceutical grade natural ingredient.

Part of our book, Defining Moments tells the story of how we left our corporate careers and began to work in the development of high performance corporate teams focused on a common cause. This ultimately led us to work with some amazing teams at some very amazing companies. Not the least of these was our time working with a number of product teams at Pfizer. There, we contributed by learning what this company with a rich history was all about. Gaining fame and fortune by developing an antibiotic that saved countless lives during World War II, Pfizer's core belief was and is the development of products designed to solve the problems people experience. Some as life threatening as Cancer and others as simple as allergy relief, the common thread is the care and concern for the quality of peoples' lives. This experience taught us much. For me, I learned that it was the quality and quantity of ingredients that would make a difference. This became a core tenant of our products and how I would solve Wendy's skin problems. It was clear to me. Simple recipes made from natural pharmaceutical grade ingredients in therapeutic proportions and without the chemical preservatives and glycols that made it easier for chemists to make products but were obviously causing many of the problems.

The idea of creating a skincare company that would make people feel good and solve their problems was still not in my mind. That would come later from my dear friend in the UK, Brian Blanchard.

200 experimental formulas to build a soap that would work for Wendy found a simple castile like soap that had a lower pH, cleaning ingredients and also included some simple oils from faraway lands suggested by some very smart new found aboriginal friends also reversed Wendy's skin conditions. This new soap coupled with a lotion made from natural oils using a process my grandmother used to make her own lotion in a pot simmering over the pilot light of her gas stove became Wendy's regime to recovery.

My friend Brian, visiting on business from the UK used the soap in our guest shower and noted that it was good, but I needed to do something about the label. I personally thought that the clear plastic bottle with a Sharpie hand written "Spa Rx" was perfectly good. This small British humor comment sparked the beginning of our company.

More and more people began to use our products and comment about how they worked to solve some seeming unsolvable problems they or their family was having. This inspired us to start sending out small sample bottles to people and on those occasions where we were offsite with one of the Pfizer teams, we would hand them samples to try. It was one of our high level executive friends at Pfizer who said to us, "You should checkout this database called Skin Deep created by this group called the EWG."

The comment by our friend at Pfizer was indeed another defining moment for us and our not yet created company. Through our investigations, we decided to make a go of creating a company that was focused on making skincare products to make people feel good and solve their problems.

For us the first step was to try to find a trade show to attend and exhibit our products just to see if anyone would care enough to part with their money to try our products. We discovered the Natural Products Expo and called them to see if we could exhibit at their show scheduled for just a few months away. Laughing, the salesperson told us that she would put us on the wait list for the show four years from now, undeterred, we decided to test market our products in Key West Florida. A favorite home away from home for us, the Florida Keys embody one of the most no nonsense diverse markets where we could test our products without the benefit of the tradeshow. During our visit, the phone rang and a person on the other end said that they were from Expo East and that someone had cancelled their booth in the personal care section. Were we interested...Yes! And this marked yet another defining moment for our idea.

We attended the Expo. One week before, our company description was due for publication in the tradeshow catalog addendum. What would be our name? No kidding, we really did not have a company name. Funny, we used the name Keys on the test market bottles, but that was because we were there testing, but Keys it was. I recall Wendy saying, Coke and Keys. Both are a consonant and are one syllable. Must be a good sign, she said.

Next question for the addendum, your tagline…We thought and thought and came up with, Chemical-Free Skin Health. That said it all for us. Little did we know that it would drive a number of people at the Expo insane! We described our products as skincare that helped to solve skin problems and made people feel good because they had a few simple natural pharmaceutical grade ingredients in therapeutic proportions. Further, we said, they contain no parabens, glycols or any of the other "Dirty Dozen" ingredients that were being promoted by the Marin County Cancer projects as leading to elevated Cancer rates in their area.

We stood in our booth realizing that we were pretty far back from the tradeshow entrance. I remember sharing with Wendy, "If it is anything like high tech, we might see our first visitor in an hour or two." We made sure we would be ready when they arrived. When the announcement came that the show was open, we were mobbed in the first few minutes. Not by the tradeshow attendees, but by the exhibitors, their formulators and scientists. I spent the entire first day answering questions and the word spread quickly that we were showing a chemical-free sunblock prototype in the booth. By the second day, scientists and chemists from the likes of Schering-Plough and others flew in to ask questions about how we stabilized the products, achieved homogenous concentrations and dispersion of uncoated zinc oxide and why oh why would we have chosen nano zinc oxide when everyone knew that it was harmful?

My answer then as it is now is that I use science and engineering to develop our products and that if they could provide me with research to show me why something is harmful or will not work that I would love to read it. Many years later now, no one has handed me anything scientific to read….only articles written by non-scientists attempting to create Fear Uncertainly and Doubt- FUD as we called it in high tech!

We started a website thinking that we would sell a few products over the web. Wendy's background at Coca-Cola was fertile training as the world's most recognized brand. We thought, we are self-funded and not impatient. The experience with the retailers at the Expo show was equally disappointing because most would ask what distributor we were going to use and countless brokers told us that we would have to follow the pattern established by the industry or we would not survive. Basically, the old child's game of a bunch of people standing around saying, "one for me, one for me, one for me and none for you." Yes, by the time we added up all the discounts, commissions and payouts, subtracting our manufacturing costs, there was nothing left for us. Worse, according to them, the higher cost of our ingredients thrust us well above the average shelf price of the industry, they said. It did not matter that our products were designed to solve problems, what was important was the label, bottle and the fragrance. I exclaimed that these are natural medicines and are one-third the price of prescription products that almost work. They did not care, they were right and we were wrong!

We left the tradeshow, not angry, but empowered that we would create an online business that made and designed products for people with chemical based skin disorders, those with sensitive skin and for Cancer recovery patients. We were very happy and set off to build our factory, make our products and to list them on that Skin Deep report. We really did not care what people thought, because I was battle worn from the PC wars in the early 80's and Wendy had gone toe-to-toe with the likes of Pepsi. The Expo was nice, but seemed like 'mouse nuts,' to us in the bigger scheme of things.

The next few months found our business growing by word of mouth and we could see our investment being returned to us in short order. Our sunblock was now on the market in time for summer. Even though our sunblock is a cosmetic everyday product for the face, neck and hands, we knew that people are more sun conscious in the summer, so we completed the move to our new factory just as the season broke. Months earlier, we had filled out all the forms to be added to the Skin Deep report and frankly had completely forgotten about it. We were so busy that we also did not notice that someone in New York had ordered ten bottles of our Solar Rx sunblock. Later we found out that it was not for one person, it was for Consumer Reports Magazine.

In the heat of the summer season, our products appeared on the Skin Deep report. We had no idea except for the fact that our orders doubled. We were ranked number one safest products in our categories on the report...amazing! Then in early July, Consumer Reports magazine ranked Solar Rx the number 1 most effective cosmetic sunscreen testing for both UVA and UVB protection. Also holding us up in a sidebar article as, "the only company telling the truth" in regard to nano particles. After all we knew they were really safe because of all the scientific studies. What could be the big deal?

Over the past years, we have continued to support the movement and efforts of the EWG (Environmental Working Group) and SafeCosmetics.org not because of their controversial positions, but because we see them helping people through education and understanding. And with all the history of our company and products offered only as background, Chemical-Free Skin Health® is a book to support this educational effort.

This book is for you! My hope is that I will have provided some foundation, common sense, and simple logic to help you form an opinion of what is right for you and more important, what is wrong for you. Truly, natural products can help you and hurt you as well if you are not careful. Those chemists working for those big companies are not the bad guys, they believe in what they are doing is right. The question? Are they right for you?

We all have choices in life. Directions we can take caused by defining moments. Our course was altered by Cancer and I have some strong opinions. These are my truths. With a small 't' because they are mine. They are not the solemn Truth because none of us really know for sure what is right or wrong in the bigger picture over time. What I offer is my perspective on things right now and what I see going on in this Chemical-Free Skin Health war between the natural players and those supporting 'more and more is less'.

When I first revealed this book at a Safe Cosmetics Compact Signer meeting at Expo West in California an individual said. "what gives you the right to write a book like this, you are not a chemist." My answer, "Exactly that reason and why don't you wait to read it before taking shots? After all, then you can write a book about my book and I promise to read yours!"

If you have not already detected it, I do not take myself too seriously. Even though this is a very important subject and at a sensitive time in the history of personal care, I feel that we cannot make knee jerk reactions. Here, I will try to give you my perspective of things as lightly as I can possibly can. This is only one man's view, albeit a man with some pretty powerful scientific resources at his disposal and some very bright minds of my friends from around the world.

Bob Root, Keys Technologist

An unlikely formulator!

Chapter 2: Weird Science or Wired Scientist

The definition of insanity is doing same thing the same way and expecting a different result!

Bob Root

To understand this book, you have to understand me. That is certainly a tall order, because I do not understand me. I think it is worth a glimpse into the mind of "One of the crazy ones!"

I am curious and a problem solver that believes that every situation is unique. Every new problem begins with a clean slate. Experience reminds me of what I have done, but does not direct me. New answers come from new thinking. I stand on the shoulders of the brightest minds that I can find. Although controversy is the number 1 tool of marketing, science dictates the direction of engineering.

Even though I believe chemists add and engineers subtract, we are on the same mission. Our mission is to make people lives better.

There is a picture of me, at the age of four, kneeling with my head on the floor looking sideways while my puppy ate his food. Was I curious about eating or just trying to figure out how the dog worked. Probably both and I have stayed that way ever since.

I have always taken things apart to see how they worked. Recently, I have figured out how to put them back together.

Yes, curious is a good word and as a scientist, I must add the phrase, "without being judgmental." I truly believe that everyone contributes.

Even the people that think I am one of the crazy ones! I am honored because of the company I am included in.

I am naturally mischievous. Once around the age of five, I climbed onto my father's workbench, snagged the biggest screwdriver I could find and proceeded to go around the neighborhood removing license plates and switching them on all the cars on my street. Still do not know why, but it still seems funny to me.

Up until recently, I received, read and kept every Popular Science Magazine for as long as I can remember. Now I read it online.

Most of my interest from early school years was both the cosmos and the world of the small. I studied the teachings of a guy named Mandelbrot who believed that the world of the sub-atomic, nano, micro and macro worlds all are the same, just a different size. One just smaller than the other and predictable because of that reality. I now contribute to the Mandelbrot Julia Chain theory by working in the quantum world.

In high school, I learned that I was a fledgling member of the Crazy Ones because I was really different. I was fascinated by the Disney Imagineers while my friends followed local sports teams. When my high school sweetie's dad asked me what I wanted to do after college, I said I wanted to be an Audio Animatronics engineer working for Disney. He had a puzzled look about him. I would still like to do that, but my world was changed suddenly. I had to join the real world of finding a real career or so I was told.

Most of my career has also been in the world of the small. I guess you can say that I am a small thinker!

My experience with working with Polaroid instant film for scientific purposes led me to an understanding of regular pure patterns created on surfaces to provide high-resolution images. Somewhat similar in understanding how similar shaped objects can self assemble to provide maximum UV protection in a sunblock. My work with Holograms began to make me think in the digital world where nothing is lost.

Later, I was lured to the new world of synthetic imaging in California. The early beginnings of what is now Lucas Film saw the rise of computers creating synthetic images that we now call digital animation or virtual reality. Applying what I learned in these early days was that all of what we were doing bucked the conventional way of thinking. Indirectly it taught me persistence and believing in myself. This is a trait that served me well in bucking the conventional thinking in both the natural and conventional skincare marketplace.

I have been sort of an entrepreneur as long as I can remember. Figuring out something to make for a particular holiday to sell to the neighbors or figuring out how to invent a better 'fuzz' box for psychedelic guitarists was more about the challenge than the money. Walking that different path always was very lonely, but I rather liked being alone. It sure beat hard core competition. Being different was differentiations for me and the things I made. You can recognize me on the street because I do not follow the trends. Maybe I am just oblivious in my small thinking world.

In the early 1980's this place called Silicon Valley caught my attention. The world of the PC was full of contenders while IBM's PC division was the gorilla in the bathroom. The idea of wearing a white shirt, black skinny tie, a pen pocket protector and looking like everyone else just did not fit me. So you guessed it, I hung with the Apple Macintosh group, wore a ratty t-shirt and thought small. Thinking in the world of small, I gravitated to data storage. While working with Polaroid, we figured out how to put spots on an instant film and read them digitally to create WORM media (Write Once Read Many). This aligning of data points again influenced my thinking about how a sunblock should self-assemble into a smooth blocking surface.

Over time, I was involved with much of the innovation in data storage. Whether it was tape, optical or hard disks, I rose up in the valley to that fateful day where I was promoted to CEO of a publically traded company. What that meant to me was that I could no longer play in the lab, I served the shareholders more than my team and I could never quite figure out what I was really supposed to be doing. All this time moving so fast and sure that I did not realize that the corporate bad guys were chasing me until I quit. As they metaphorically shot by me when I put on the career brakes, I remember having the conversation with Wendy as she simultaneously resigned from Coke and wondering what this was all about. We were both somewhat amazed that our careers were so focused on the ambition and challenges that we never had time to look in the rear view mirror. Ironically, this still serves us today as the world of natural products undergoes transformation and a strange sort of concern for what people think versus what is right.

In our team consulting business, I wanted to understand how people think. No, not a typo. Not what people think, but how they think! Being a geek, I turned to other geeks like Marvin Minsky (Minsky's Mind author) and two cats from UC Santa Cruz named Bandler and Grinder. The three were working on a similar project to create new software that would operate the way people think. Minsky at MIT had mapped the neural process and the Santa Cruz cats had figured out the concept called Neuro Linguistic Programming (NLP). NLP mapped how people communicated meaning through Visual, Auditory and Kinesthetic means. So, Wendy and I studied and trained in NLP and my particular study area became refined in a sector called NLP timelines. Time lining is the study of looking at the past trajectory and determining future trends and direction. As a sub facet, it helped me recognize that people predominately communicate meaning visually and then through feelings. In the bigger scheme of things, not only am I a small thinker, but I learned that I am dominate auditory, a little less visual and absolutely zero kinesthetic. At least I thought.

Most of my life, most of my friends would tell you that I am not a touchy feely sensitive sort of guy. Wendy jokes that when we first met in Santa Fe that she was trying to get my attention as I ate at breakfast the day we first met. Her version is funnier, but it took a kick from one of my engineers, Simon, and an alert that this great looking babe across the table was trying to get my attention. She did thanks to a bruised shin from Simon. So, I used to not be a very sensitive guy.

There have been only a few things that have knocked my legs out from underneath me. Wendy's Cancer was one of them. Getting through the surgery and recovery, my soft underbelly was really exposed watching this lifelong beauty suffer from all sorts of skin disorders post-surgery. Once a golden tanned blond haired beauty, she was still beautiful to me pale and marked with things that looked like eczema one day, psoriasis the next and then adult acne. We would sit at meeting and I would watch her unconsciously scratch at her neck trying to think through a problem. Only to notice giant welts appearing in a few seconds. She would run to the rest room to apply a prescription ointment that would miraculously knock it down only to find redness and irritation a few hours later. It was breaking my heart because it was breaking Wendy's. She had beaten Cancer, but could not beat the chemicals in the products designed to help her. Equally, as she used more of them, she needed more and stronger prescriptions because the old ones stopped working. Clearly I did not realize her sensitivity emotionally and when I connected the dots that it was the chemicals in the products meant to help her and how her emotions were being frayed because of them I really got pissed.

This was the start of Keys, but more important, I have had five years of her improved skin health and meeting hundreds of people that suffer like her. But it was a letter from a woman sent through our customer service group that woke me up again sparking me to pickup and finish this book I started two years ago.

She wrote, "I have scratched my skin until it bleeds for ten years! Doctor after doctor prescribed lotion and serums to get me to stop this terrible affliction. I searched for any alternative and discovered Keys through the Safe Cosmetics (Skin Deep) Report . I went to your website and read the story of the woman that Wendy helped that sounded just like my affliction. Mickey (Keys Customer Service), you reminded me that it was the cause that was important to figure out and not just a product to fix the symptoms. You reminded me to check my laundry detergent and I suddenly realized that like the woman, I was washing my bedding everyday with a questionable product. I bought new sheets and only washed them in simple soap. Within two weeks, my itching and scratching was gone. I realized that I was cured after ten years. I was and am so appreciative that my life has changed and my outlook is again one that is positive. Another part of me is angry and wondered how our government can allows this sort of thing to happen to me. Then it hit me with such a force. I am in charge of me and my life. I just didn't understand what was going on. Thanks to you I now do! "

I shared the story with a friend who is a makeup artist and self-proclaimed health nut. When I commented that the woman should understand, she blasted me by telling me that "just because you know this stuff does not mean the rest of us do." I retorted, "I am not an expert only an observer and that I am an unlikely unqualified formulator." "So then tell people what you think and let them make up their minds, she said!" So, now I am!

Chapter Tools

1. The personal care industry is dynamic and changes daily.

2. Research and accumulate information daily.

3. Follow your intuition about products, doctors, people, companies and trends.

4. Listen to people for what they are saying, meaning and feeling.

5. You need to go first when it comes to protecting yourself and your family.

6. You do not have to be an expert to know what is right for you.

As a lifelong student of linguistics, I realize that we use words, our tone of voice and our body language to communicate meaning to others. Meaning is an interesting word because it carries with it some history, the present and the future. Words can inspire or create fear. They can make us feel secure and raise us to action.

When I chose to write this book and choose its title, part of my decision was from all the negativity surrounding the industry. It seems to me that it is sort of a war between conventional chemists and natural compounders. There have been tons of things written about what is wrong. I found very little written about what is right.

Think about it! How many times have you had someone ask you 'what's wrong?' How many times have people asked you, "What's Right?" I know it sounds funny, but the words of safety and harm are similar. Often we confuse them and sometimes even invert them. Do two negatives make a positive?

On our website for our products, we exclaim No SLS, No Parabens and use the term Chemical-Free as a tag line almost as the antithesis of Better Living Through Chemistry. My reality is that what we want to achieve is safety for our customers and educate them without operating from a place of fear. Yet, it bothers me that we lead with No this and No that.

In my interaction with people all over the world at a one-on-one level, I have the opportunity to listen and learn. When I first meet people, I find myself asking what is important to them when it comes to themselves and their family. It is a funny thing, because when I ask the question, my intent is about the skin health. Interestingly, they usually answer based on their lives.

Safety is always paramount and takes on various forms based on age and where people live in the world. For example, 60+ people will often say "my home" meaning shelter. Boomers will often say security, meaning financial security. Gen-X I hear saying "safety" meaning physical security and Gen-Y/Nexters the term seems to be a freedom from all of the things of the past.

To me and in the context of this book, the word safe means many things as well. We do not often think of safety in terms of time. Is it going to hurt me right now is the typical meaning. Will something hurt me over time or will it harm my children are normally reserved for conflicts between nations, financial situations or genetic health issues. We seem to assume that someone in the government, our doctors or some voiceless guardian will protect us from the food we eat or the products we use on our body.

What will hurt me, harm me, age me or shorten my life...

There are so many books about what can harm you. I read the chemical list called the Dirty Thirty produced by the organizational offshoot of Search for the Cause, called Teens Turning Green (www.TeensTurningGreen.com) and I applaud them for their compilation of some very questionable chemicals used widely in the personal care and cosmetics industry. The Environmental Working

Group database report called Skin Deep (www.safecosmetics.org) that ranks product safety and details on both chemical and natural ingredients. The Compact for Safe Cosmetics aligns manufacturers to create products that do not use toxic chemicals. And the Breast Cancer Fund for focusing on chemicals that are suspected of causing this terrible form of Cancer. Clearly some of the chemicals used in skin care and cosmetics are very toxic, but there are other things that are unsafe that are natural.

Lead is natural, but does not belong in lipstick and it is in most lipsticks. Silica is perhaps the most commonly used element to produce glass and computer chips. Yet, in its raw state ground into a fine powder and inhaled can cause silicosis and is considered a carcinogen. Some chemicals in products carry a safety term called GRAS meaning "generally accepted as safe," because they have been used for a long time. Is ten years a long time or is 100 years a long time. Since it sometimes takes thousands of years to mutate a species, what happens when you shock the body by adding chemicals that never existed?

Harm to me is a much broader term. If we remove the protective mantle of the skin chemically and then microorganisms attack, or bacteria attack or a fungus, the harm is indirect and yet still harmful. When we use an anti-bacterial soap, our hands are clean and germ-free. The soap itself does no direct harm, but it can open the door to infection from staph, fungus or other diseases.

Microbiology is such a concern to me that is perhaps more immediately threatening than toxic chemicals. When we "go natural," and "chemical-free," we are indirectly saying that we are avoiding chemicals originally designed to help protect us. Parabens in products are ingredients because they were designed to kill bacteria to protect us. The generalized belief is that they do a great job in the bottle, but harm us when that ingredient comes in contact with our skin. Yes, I find it sometimes unbelievable that people that I talk to actually believe that the germicides and bactericides used in products do not disappear when they come out of the bottle. What makes then affective in killing bad things in the bottle also keep going when they come in contact with our skin. Hurt the bacteria on our skin and you harm us. It is that simple.

The argument for bactericides and other anti-fungal or germicides is a strong one when you compare it to the power of some gram negative and gram positive bacteria. Staph infections, E.coli and other microbiology-based attackers are terrifying and can be deadly. That is why our food is prepared a certain way, then protected by processes and finally tested to be free of bacteria that can harm us. While cheeses and penicillin gain their benefits from bacteria colonies, other colonies of bacteria can harm us and have to be reviewed.

Perceptions that low doses of certain chemicals is not harmful often surprises me in a world of science where we discover every day about residual chemicals, hormone and even radiation embed in our cells and tissue. These small doses adding up to become toxic is simply science and are easy to detect if you are looking for them. Studies time and again find industrial chemicals in the placenta from new born babies. These industrial chemicals have been tracked to water supplies, the materials that construct our homes and those chemicals in our environment. A hand full of teens agreed to have their blood tested for chemicals, well known reporters have done the same. Authors and TV show producers have also submitted to testing. All are a little different, but all found hundreds of chemicals present in their body. I believe the teens had over 300 chemicals that were found, but also found hormones, antibiotics and steroids. All of which they did not take, but were present.

Toxic and heavy metals are a growing concern with numerous types of these metals embedding themselves in our bodies and building up over time.

Antibacterial biocides that we use to clean our hands that destroy all of the natural safe guarding bacteria on our skin and worse are now used in foods to preserve them to make them safe. At the same time is the bactericide in the plastic wrap on that cheese we just bought (that preserves the product so that we can buy a bigger slice to save money) the same bactericide that researchers believe are killing the probiotic in our gut. Fact or fiction? Cause and effect?

Some of the beauty regimes literally burn our skin off claiming that they are natural acids from apples and will help us.

People use Ultraviolet C (UVC) rays to bleach, treat and modify the skin for beauty sake not thinking that we are exposing ourselves to potentially disfiguring collagen destruction. They use the same UVC light to sterilize our countertops and yet the lamp used in a factory requires protective goggles and clothing.

Safety to me is both short term and long-term consequence.

Stop, Challenge and Choose!

I chose this as a subtitle for this book because it is both the call to action and because it is the best way I know of when confronting fears, concerns or worry. Harm is often averted if we Stop, Challenge and Choose. Making the right decisions is imperative with the really big things in our lives. So it is true if we use the practice for the small things that can harm us over time or even indirectly. It does take a change in thinking and reacting.

What Stop Challenge Choose means is that when you are confronted with something that triggers feelings, doubt or concern, stop everything, challenge what is in front of you and choose the appropriate direction for you.

Stop, Challenge and Choose can be understood with a simple example of walking up to a busy intersection with no traffic light. Fear of being hit by a car stops you. You challenge the need to get across the street by studying and noticing a traffic light a block away. Taking you no farther away from your destination, you choose to continue to cross at the traffic light. Making the same choices about the food and diet you choose is the same as the products you use on your skin. Like crossing where there is no light, unknowingly using products on your skin is just as dangerous.

Worrying is also toxic. It would be so nice to live in a truly safe world where the products we use on our skin are all healthy for us. So even though there are literally thousands of blogs, websites and opinions out there, to me the message is clear. For the safety of yourself, your family, your pets and friends, I want you to go forward with one single belief. That is to Stop, Challenge and Choose what feels right for you after in depth research. It is important to understand what makes sense for you and not someone else.

Follow your intuition about people, products and companies. Think of your intuition as a compilation of what you have learned in your life, what you were taught and what you think, feel, see and hear. Roll all of the possible data sources into your emotional mind knowing that the decisions you make can and should be simple steps testing your intuitional footing as you go.

Some may find this chapter confusing. For others, you might find it as a new way of looking at things. Others may realize that they have started to understand that they are on the right track.

The over-arching message is that you have to take responsibility for your own safety. Clearly, this book will have succeeded if you now have an understanding that what you put on your body in the form of cosmetics and personal care products may harm you.

Chapter Tools

1. Safety is personal and means something different to everyone.

2. There are many aspects of personal care and cosmetics products that may harm you short and long term.

3. Understanding what can harm you, your family, your pets and friends takes study to form your intuition. The smarter you are the stronger your intuition.

4. The secret to safety is to Stop, Challenge and Choose a direction based on information from many sources.

5. Think of your intuition as your emotional mind making decisions based on input, action and reaction.

6. Sorry, there is no one watching over you as an individual.

7. Do not assume that because a product you use has a barcode that it means that it is safe and tested. It probably has not been tested.

Chapter 4: Skin Game or Skin Health

This book is about the skin, but with a hard twist. The real question is who is controlling what goes on our skin? If you trust the manufacturer then they do. If you become your own guardian and be responsible for what you use, then you need some tools. Albeit a friendly war between chemical products and their natural counterparts, it is a war none-the-less. It is a friendly war because manufacturers will respond to what you want. If you sit quietly, they listen to the few and themselves. If you speak up, you will be heard. Until the trend turns, it is indeed chemicals versus the natural alternatives.

Much of what this book is about is balance. It is a balance between the flora on our skin and the products that we use that sometimes can destroy the very fabric of our skin.

I struggled for an analogy for the balance of the skin with our environment.

The human body contains 10 times as many bacterial cells as it does human cells.

Scientists have found that the bacteria that live on our skin are extraordinarily diverse. The bacteria around our eyes are different from the nose, just a few centimeters away. So is true of the bacteria on our arms, the creases at our elbows and behind the ear. Our bacteria are a biosphere on our skin.

Researchers at Columbia University did tests sampling twenty different spots on the body and found an extreme variation in type and form. What they began to map is that different bacteria were associated with different areas on the body and they had different disorders associated with these areas.

The Balance of the Skin

Researchers have wondered for some time why eczema is always inside the elbow and psoriasis is on the outside of the elbow. Those human cells are the same. As close as the inside and outside are together, the microbes that live inside the elbow and outside the elbow are uniquely different. Psoriasis and eczema do not appear to be caused by bacteria, but they could be a reaction, triggered by a change in the ecosystems of germs on our skin.

My personal belief in reading all the literature and research is that the balance of microbes, to skin cell type, to fungus and bacteria on the body may be the cause. As troubling as these simple disorders are to people, we still do not have the cause, but I believe scientists are close. Our customers using some of our products have told us that they have seen relief to reversal, but truth be told, we still do not know why.

How Bacteria Affect Us

And skin is just the start. The National Institutes of Health is now embarking on a follow-up to the human genome project, called the Human Microbiome Project.

A researcher at the Human Genome Project was quoted in an NPR article as saying, "The human genome is really an amalgamation of the human cells and the bacterial cells," she says, "and it's time for us to turn attention to the other organisms that live together with our human cells."

Given the enormous variety of bacteria that she has cataloged with this latest census, it's likely that the bacteria in total have far more genes than we do. It will be a challenge to decipher them all, but that's the goal."

The best analogy that I can come up with that will help you realize the impact of bacteria and the balance of the skin is as simple as the air we breathe.

So, throughout this book hold in your thoughts the following belief I have:

"The bacteria on our skin are like the atmosphere that surrounds the earth." It protects us, it serves us and it holds a balance that must be maintained.

Skin 101

Ironically, in preparing for this book, I realized how much I did not know about the skin. OK, you say that I should being in the business, but I am being honest. I literally spent 50+ hours reading and barely scratched the surface of the world's knowledgebase. What was even more shocking is that when I talked to many skincare professionals, I found that they even knew less than I did. Worse, many felt they knew more than they really did. And these are the people that are supposed to know that we as inquiring minds want to be assured of their knowledge. I assume that if I did not know the things I learned and that the professionals I talked to were less informed than me, then I can only assume that the average person knows less. This is the reason for this section and its proximity to the front of the book.

You can think of the following as a refresher if you already knew all of what I am about to explain.

Our Magical Skin Exposed

The skin is one of the most important components of our physical appearance and is the largest organ of our body. It fulfills many functions that support our lives physically and are the sole contributor to the attraction between people. If you have bad skin, it alters your self-esteem. Conversely having great skin attracts.

The skin does offer us many functions. In fact, it may have the most functions of any of our other organs. Organ you say? Yes, the skin is our largest organ. I know I have said this, but before reading on, please grasp the magnitude of this largest organ of ours.

Here are some of the things our skin does.

1. The skin protects our internal structures from injury. Think of it as a flexible membrane that pads our other organs against injury.
2. The skin protects against external bacteria and viruses. This will become even more an important function as more toxins are thrown upon us in the form of pollution and chemicals. It is also important when we consider using anti-bacterial products that indiscriminately kill good and bad bacteria.

3. The skin exchanges fluids and gases from our body into the environment. This includes oxygen and CO2 as well as water in the form of perspiration.

4. The skin is the number one organ responsible for regulating our temperature by regulating blood flow and sweat.

5. The skin also protects us from UV radiation by forming melanin to darken the skin and offer protection form UVA and UVB rays. Of course, we all should know that 90% of visible skin aging comes from UV and skin Cancer is on the rise because we have abused this facet of the skin. More about this later.

6. The skin also acts as an immune organ to detect infections. Yes, we see the results of our health on our skin. That is why doctors of the past looked us over head-to-toe before an exam. Scientists have been able to detect breast Cancer using thermal imaging. I think you get the picture.

7. The skin acts as a sensory organ to detect temperature, touch and vibration. Here I want you to think about those chemicals we are going to talk about and how they could change how the skin functions. Just maybe those chemicals in some sunscreens that make us sweat profusely could be altering the way the skin receptors detect what temperature is correct.

8. My favorite is that the skin functions as visible signal for social and sexual communication. Does that bride really glow? Yes she does. This fact is one of the secrets to what I am calling New Beauty!

There are many more purposes of the skin and worth a few minutes to Google when you get a chance. For me and the rest of the point of this book, these are the eight most important to me.

Our skin is a naturally evolved organ that can deal with many gradual changes over time. Things like huge rises in pollution or other environmental occurrences like chemicals coming in contact with it do not permit the skin to evolve fast enough. So the skin can do only one thing. React! This is a key point as we explore skin disorders. Are they genetic, maybe! Can they be caused by external factors? Definitely!

The skin is the outer covering of the body. In humans, it is the largest organ of the body's integrity system and has multiple layers of tissue. It guards muscles, the bones and internal organs.

Because it interfaces with the environment, skin plays a key role in protecting the body against pathogens and excessive water loss.

It also functions as an insulator, temperature regulation, sensation, synthesis of vitamin D, and the protection of vitamin B. Severely damaged skin will try to heal by forming scar tissue. This is often discolored and the pigment is lost.

Skin pigmentation varies among populations, and skin type can range from dry to oily. Such skin variety provides a rich and diverse habit for bacteria that number roughly at 1000 species.

Skin has mesoderm cells, pigmentation provided by melanin, which absorb some of the dangerous ultraviolet radiation (UVA and UVB) in sunlight. It also contains DNA-repair enzymes that help reverse UV damage, and people who lack the genes for these enzymes suffer high rates of skin Cancer.

One form of this genetic deficiency is produced by UV light. Malignant melanoma, which my wife Wendy had, is particularly invasive, causing it to spread quickly, and can often be deadly.

Human skin pigmentation varies among populations in a wide band. This has led to the classification of people on the basis of skin color. It has been, in fact, the reason for wars, discrimination and classification. Does skin color matter? Yes, and hopefully less and less because it really does not matter!

The skin is the largest organ in the human body. For the average adult human, the skin has a surface area of between 15 square feet and 21 square feet. The skin is an average thickness of about 0.1 inches. The average square inch of skin holds 650 sweat glands, 20 blood vessels, 60,000 melanin cells, and more than 1,000 nerve endings.

Skin performs the following functions:

Protection: an anatomical barrier from pathogens and damage between the internal and external environment in bodily defense. The skin is part of the adaptive immune system.

The sensation capability of skin stems from a variety of nerve endings that react to heat and cold, touch, pressure, vibration, and tissue injury.

In heat regulation, the skin contains a blood supply far greater than its requirements that allows precise control of energy loss by radiation, convection and conduction. Dilated blood vessels increase perfusion and heat loss, while constricted vessels greatly reduce blood flow and conserve heat.

Controlling evaporation, the skin provides a relatively dry and semi-impermeable barrier to fluid loss. Loss of this function contributes to the massive fluid loss in burns.

Concerning attraction esthetics and communication, others see our skin and can assess our mood, physical state and attractiveness.

The skin also acts as a storage center for lipids and water, as well as a means of synthesis of vitamin D by action of UV on certain parts of the skin.

Sweating contains urea. Even though this is a small amount, keeping the skin clean helps remove this natural toxin. Continuing the thought, we want to clean our skin and not disinfect it.

Absorption is perhaps one of the most understudied and overlooked functions of the skin. In addition, medicine can be administered through the skin, by ointments or by means of adhesive patch, such as the nicotine patch or weight loss remedies. So, as drugs and medicines go, so goes the chemicals we are exposed to everyday in the form of pollutants and products we put on our skin.

Not the least of the interesting facets of the skin is its water resistance. The easiest way I like to describe this part of the function of the skin is it is like Gore-Tex®. The skin breathes and it is water tight as well as water resistant. This facet is why I do not make a waterproof sunblock for the entire body.

Skin care

The skin supports its own ecosystems of microorganisms, including yeasts and bacteria, which cannot be removed by any amount of cleaning. That said, it could be destroyed by chemicals. Parabens and Triclosan used in antibacterial sanitizers have been shown to break down this defense system. Study on this is still too young, but following the principle of Occam's Razor, the simple and most obvious answer is probably true. Estimates place the number of individual bacteria on the surface of one square inch of human skin at 50 million. Oily surfaces, such as the face, may contain over 500 million bacteria per square inch. This is why the face is acne prone. Interestingly, the various microorganisms on the skin tend to keep each other in balance unless chemicals and UVA are introduced. Yes, those UVC lights kill bacteria the same way that parabens and Triclosan type chemicals do. Throwing these bacteria out of balance is what I believe is the cause of many skin disorders. When the balance is disturbed, there may be an overgrowth and infection, such as when antibiotics kill microbes, resulting in an overgrowth of yeast. I believe that any time we kill bacteria, whether it is to get rid of acne or exfoliate our skin, we are exposing our skin and our body to infiltration by even worse bacteria strains like staph, MRSA or E.coli infections.

Proper skin hygiene is important because unclean skin favors the development of pathogenic organisms. The dead cells that continually slough off the epidermis mix with the secretions of the sweat and sebaceous glands and the residual on the skin form a layer on its surface. If not washed away, the slurry of sweat and sebaceous secretions mixed with dirt and dead skin is decomposed by bacterial flora, producing smell. Functions of the skin are disrupted when it is excessively dirty; it becomes more easily damaged, the release of antibacterial compounds decreases and dirty skin is more prone to develop infections. I also believe that if we layer waterproof liquids or lotions on our skin, it exacerbates this unhealthy effect. You may have heard about painted models dying of skin suffocation and there have been stories about those people in the Blue Man Group managing this effect.

Cosmetics should be used carefully on the skin because these may cause allergic reactions. They may also cause suffocation in a minor form leading to deteriorated skin health. It does make me wonder. If clear clean skin is beautiful, attractive to the opposite sex and tells someone else all about us, then why do we cover it up? Maybe makeup is really covering up our feelings. Or maybe we are just hiding.

Oily Skin

Oily skin is wonderful because it is less likely to wrinkle. On the negative side, oily skin is heavy, clogs the pores, is more likely to have pimples and therefore makes us feel and look bad. That shine or glisten is not so bad compared to the alternative. The best thing to keep overact sebum from happening is a balanced skin health regime. Shock therapy in the form of harsh exfoliants, scrubs and acid washes just cause the skin to react as violently as what initially caused the reaction. That is why post these treatments our skin turns bright red. Just like in sunburn, the skin is damaged and studies have shown that the sebum reacts even more intensely. So, the message about oily skin is subtle rebalancing.

Some research contends that the best deterrent for oily skin comes from taking Vitamin B3 and/or niacin while gently cleaning the skin with slightly alkaline soaps.

Aging

Studies have shown that 90% of visible skin aging comes from UV exposure. True! Next time you jump out of the shower, look at you bum in the mirror. That is what skin that is not exposed to UV looks like.

Yes, people say, as we get older the skin thins. In addition, our diet has something to do with it. True, the chemicals we use on our skin also can affect it one way or the other. Pollution also plays a role, but remember pollution is merely an airborne chemical. Still, if 90% of all visible aging comes from the sun, all those other factors add up to only 10%. So, if we only spent as much on protecting our skin from UV, we would not need all those other things in the form of chemical based cosmetics and personal care. Do you think? ...or am I just hallucinating?

If it is not my hallucination, then the prescription for young healthy skin may be simpler than you think and would include keeping the skin clear and clean while staying out of the sun. That simple? Yes!

Chapter Tools

1. The balance on our skin is like the balance of the atmosphere that surrounds the earth.
2. Stay out of the sun!
3. Don't tan!
4. Reduce the chemical load on your skin.
5. Wash regularly and gently.
6. Let your skin go bare as often as possible.
7. If you use makeup then use it around the eyes, the cheeks and lips adding color and letting the real you show through.
8. Drink lots of water.
9. Laugh as often as possible.

Chapter 5: Chemical in Our Products...The Beginnings

"We are the reason we have more chemicals in our lives because we asked for them!"

Bob Root

I was at a store in downtown Vancouver BC Canada and a young lady was talking to me about natural skin care. Her tone was friendly and she reminded me of Wendy a bit. She did not look like her, but there was something about the way she talked about chemicals in skincare and household products that reminded me of Wendy. Then suddenly I heard the voice of Wendy's long-term girlfriend and college roommate, Linda. I remember Linda describing Wendy as "often wrong and never in doubt!" Listening to the young lady talk, more and more I heard Linda's voice. Then I realized what it was. The young woman believed that all the chemicals she was talking about have been in products forever. I stopped her and asked this simple question. Did you know that before World War II that there were almost no synthetic chemicals in our products? That just 60 years ago, most everything that we put in and on our bodies was natural?

OK, that is not totally truth, but I had to get her attention after all!

Turns out what I said was close to correct and I started to realize that most of what I was reading in internet blogs and the press sounded like the natural movement is something new and that it is full of revelations coming one by one every day. The new enlightened act as if the world has always been synthetic.

One expert shared with me that there have been more chemicals created in the last 50 years than in all of history. That the average number of ingredients in a single personal care products average 40+ chemicals compounds, while some of these compounds themselves have multiple chemicals and preservatives. Most of which have never been tested for safety.

I thought I would try to figure out when and how many of the chemicals we find in products today started. Maybe there is a connection or thread to follow. It turns out that it is very hard to track and that the safety of the chemicals is not required to be certified or tested.

What was shocking to me was that I also found that many chemicals have been renamed by their formulators creating synonyms. As the increase pressure continues on sulfates in skin and hair care as well as parabens, we are seeing companies rename these chemicals or obviously disguise them with formal Latin names called INCI (International Nomenclature of Cosmetic Ingredients) nomenclature. These are the long names you see on labels and are considered a standard by the industry.

There are varying opinions of how and when the boom in chemicals really began. My focus is on the personal care and makeup markets to see the trend beginnings and try to trace back some of the origin of when chemistry began to dominate personal care, cosmetics and household products.

In most cases the beginnings of any trend begins with an invention of a better way to do something. Often 'better way' translates to cheaper, lower cost or easier to manufacture. For example, you can buy a topical cream in the drugstore that contains cortisone for $9.95. Step to the back counter aka pharmacy, and you can pick up a prescription for prednisone for $99.95. These two topical ointments are in the same family, but one has proven over time to be easy and easier to manufacture in volume and the other is state-of-the-art of pharmacology. This is why you pay more for the prednisone and why it will be $9.95 someday. Marketers call this the adoption to volume ratio. Without having to describe in detail the Nash Manifold Theory (think the movie, A Beautiful Mind), what this theory says is that over time new products and new concepts start small and are purchased by Early Adopters. As more people buy, the Early Adopters give way to what are called Early Majority as the volume of sales rise and production ramps up. Over time and usually at the peak of a products' volume curve, the Late Majority purchase the product and as volume declines headed to zero, the Late Adopters buy the product. Somewhere around the end of the Early Adopter phase, the marketers and designers start to look to how to extend the product life cycle by adding features and revisions that customers have asked for.

So indeed, if you follow the logic, we as consumers actually set the trends and call for the next improvements and inventions.

Before I go on to describe some of the origins I found for how we began to see the rapid growth in chemicals in our personal care, cosmetics and household products, I must share a commonality that I found. In every industry sector, the products that were being used were made at home. As our society changed from rural agricultural, food began to be commoditized, packaged and made convenient. So is true of the personal care and cosmetics industry as it is true for household products.

Here is the premise. Probably the reason you are reading this book is that you are thinking about reducing your own chemical baggage, someone thinks you need to clean up your act or you are just curious.

In the above example of products being homemade moving to factory made, the emphasis moved from purpose and functionality to mass production, lower cost, more consistency and ease of purchasing.

My guess is that if you are average that you are exposing yourself to 300+ chemicals a day. That is up from just a few our ancestors that lived in the late 1800's to our parents and through to us. Reversing this trend can mean making your own, as the thousands of DIY web sites would have you believe. Yes, it is an alternative. Move to the mountains raise some goats and live off the land making your own products that you know every ingredient that goes into them...or so you think.

The reality for the other 99% of us is that we want the manufacturers to make us quality products at a fair price that will not harm us. Equally, we want to be able to buy these products at our local store. So even though the trends moved from making your own products to manufacturers making them for us, it does not mean that we have to make them ourselves. What we have to do is ask for what we want. To do that we have to know what we want.

Yes, I believe we are exposed to hundreds of chemicals daily in our lives. Worse, they are not always the same chemical each day. I started to try and figure out what these might be and realized I would need an array of thousands of chemical sniffers and a super-computer to figure it out. I must admit my manual attempt made my head hurt and I was physically depressed.

I thought of Jack Welch's quote that, "Only self-confident people can be simple." I thought, maybe only self-confident products are simple. Certainly, the corollary that complexity breeds complexity would seem to be true when it comes to cosmetics and personal care.

I got back on track and tried to figure out how all these chemicals got into our products. What I did was follow a type of product back to when it was made at home through to today in each of the three categories of cosmetics, personal care and household products.

Ironically, the paths of the three categories were almost perfectly matched for timing, amplitude and change. All three seem to make the transition from home to urban centers at the same time. The interesting thing was that from a society perspective, the convenience of having it close to where you lived did not see the rise of chemicals being used. The products were pretty much the same as they were when the people made them at home. Now they were in tins or bottles, but were fundamentally made the same way with the same natural whole ingredients.

Most of the shift that I found in personal care, cosmetics and home care moving from DIY to a factory supplier occurred in the very late 1800's through World War I. Still, the integrity of the products seemed to be intact and made the same way as their home counterparts.

The spark occurred post World War II for personal care and cosmetics. It seemed to be the scarcity of many luxury items and raw materials that were needed for War Machines that excited the chemists of the world to create synthetic versions of natural ingredients.

During World War II things like natural rubber were in short supply. Believe it or not, the invention and mass production of synthetic rubber is the focal point and defining moment of when the "big bang" of chemistry in household products, personal care and cosmetics seem to start to ever widen at uncontrollable rates.

Better Things for Better Living...Through Chemistry

In 1935 DuPont Chemical Company started using the tagline for their company. "Better Things for Better Living...Through Chemistry" stayed for many years until they dropped the Through Chemistry part. I remember as a kid hearing this phrase repeatedly on television as the company sponsored many TV shows. Even though I believe that all the synthetic ingredients created during World War II were the beginning, the real catalyst of when the personal care, cosmetics and household products began to morph, it was also the precursor to the birth of sponsored television commercials.

Looking back, I picked up a copy of the book, "Ogilvy On Advertising", written by the founder of the famous New York advertising agency, Ogilvy Mather. These guys were at the forefront of a whole new philosophy of advertising and the personal care, cosmetics and household products were at the center of their efforts. What they did was shorten the cycle of developing products by figuring out a way to test concepts of product features even before the product was even developed.

What they would do is take a product or a concept and go to stores and survey people to find out what they thought. Eventually this simple interview became a science and the entire advertising industry changed forever. This was the birth of the chemicals in our personal care products and it occurred in the 1950's through the late 1960's. Acceleration occurred after the 1970's by the wide use of bar codes shifting the demographic knowledge from the manufacturers to the stores where broad trend data could be instantly gleaned from the buying habits of people at the super market checkout. Real-Time Chemistry!

We are the Cause!

As I read all the blogs, NGO newsletters and countless chat forums seeking a new renaissance of chemical-free, I suddenly realized that we as consumers are to blame for why all the chemicals exist in products today. When someone surveys us to find out what we like in a product or dislike, it usually also has a few question of what you would like to see in future products.

These future product surveys are now in real-time because our actual buying trends are visible instantly as we buy products. For example, Clorox Toilet Bowl Cleaner has a new green version. If more of those are scanned than the conventional, that trend data is sent back to Clorox and they ramp larger production runs of the green version. So is true of the other green or conventional products sold.

In the past, when we asked for a shampoo that makes the hair feel silky or a cream rinse that detangles or both products in a large economy size, the manufacturers respond by adding sulfate, silicone and parabens. When we asked for lotions that feel the same all year round and will not melt in a hot car or freeze in the winter, manufacturers added glycols...aka chemicals.

I cannot say that I have many chemist friends, but the ones I do know are driven by trends. They do not actually sit around and think up bad things to add to products. They respond to marketing needs for whiter, brighter, smoother or better smelling products that all last longer and cost less.

If I am right and the chemistry big bang occurred prior to World War II, the universe of chemicals expanded rapidly from the invention of TV commercials blasted to a society looking for more and more convenience with little to no concern for what went into these next chemical innovations.

Chapter Tools

1. We are responsible for chemicals in products indirectly by asking for more features and benefits in products.
2. Cosmetics, personal care and household products are designed based on trends. Safer products are a trend.
3. Buy safe products and the manufacturers will make more of them.
4. Buy fewer unsafe products and manufacturers will make less of them.
5. Return products that do not work or cause a reaction or that you are afraid of. Afraid is as important as whiter, brighter to a manufacturer.
6. Read labels!

Chapter 6: The Tool Chest....You Becoming the Expert.

"The smarter you become about what you put on your body, the sooner we will all have safer products."

Bob Root

Yes, I believe this to be true now even more than any time in history. The more you know about what goes into products and the effect they may have on you the sooner manufacturers will shift their emphasis.

In the prior chapter, I talked about how the manufacturer knows instantly your buying trends from the products you purchased that are scanned and electronically sent to the manufacturers. Some know in real-time what you are buying and all know within 24 hours. Entire companies make a business of sorting these trends out and figuring what products are next. Think about it! What you buy instantly goes back to the manufacturers in the form of trend data.

So, let's say you go to the store and you buy organic food, natural toilet bowl cleaner, natural laundry detergent and a lipstick reported to have unsafe lead levels. What you send back to the manufacturer is a lot more than you think. Those bar codes told them the community you live in and because of the time of day they can guess whether you work or not. They will guess that you are female, good idea that you live with someone based on the jumbo laundry detergent you bought and that you are green conscious except for your cosmetics. If I were they, I would guess that you are interested in safer cosmetics because of all the green stuff you bought, but just unaware of the big Environmental Working Group Lead in Lipsticks report.

In this chapter, I will do my best to arm you with some simple tools that will help you to make more educated buying decisions. More choices through a broader knowledge of how to read labels, understand ingredients and deciphering the language of personal care manufacturers.

Most important take away from this chapter is that your buying trends combined with those of others sets a trend that manufacturers follow. Buy greener cleaner products and so goes the industry. Don't believe me? Five years ago, you had to go to the health food natural market to buy anything organic. Now it is available in every grocery store in even the smallest towns.

Statistically, the fastest growing segment of cosmetics and personal care is the natural segment. Why, because you are buying natural more and more.

It's Time to Get Wise

The first step in getting chemical wise in your cosmetics, personal care and household products is to learn what to look for, when to question and when to say no!

In this chapter, I want to help you understand how to read a product label and what some of the terminology of the industry is so that you can make better judgments on products.

The most important part of a product is its ingredients. There are two things to consider about ingredients:

1. What do the ingredients do or why are they in the product? and...

2. What will they do for me? The reverse is true as well...what will they do to me.

First things first! What are safe chemicals and which are not? If I listed all the chemicals that are suspected of being unsafe, it would fill a book and the list would be outdated before this book was published. So rather than identifying all the chemicals, instead my choice is to teach you how to hunt.

There are a number of resources to seek out chemical concerns. These include very sophisticated databases created by the US Government, the EU and Non Governmental Organizations (NGOs). Resources that you should not use are product company websites or blogs unless backed with footnotes of scientific studies. There are tons of opinions out there and opinions are worth what you pay for them...Nothing!

First Rule: No Ingredients...No Buy

This is my first rule that I tell people when I am in a store doing a demo or when speaking to people about skin health.

Would you buy a prepared meal or a can of food that had no ingredients on the label? I hope not. Because of my MSG reaction, I have to read every label and I am scared off when I see one that says "No MSG Added".

Simply put, if a product does not have ingredients on the label do not buy it.

Second Rule: If you cannot pronounce the ingredients on the label, research before you buy!

Big Words Can Mean Big Chemicals

There is a great deal of controversy in the industry around using the common or Latin name for products. This is called the INCI (pronounced "INKY") name. INCI again stands for International Nomenclature of Cosmetic Ingredients. This is a database available to look up common ingredients like Aloe Vera and find its INCI name which is **Aloe** Barbadensis. In this case, the INCI name is similar to the common name of Aloe Vera. Unfortunately, this is not true for most ingredients used in products today.

Later, I will tell my story of surveying Expo West industry experts as to what the real names were for ten ingredients presented to them by their INCI names. Because most could not answer the survey correctly, some in the industry realized and changed direction. This and other movements in the industry lead to listing both names on a label. So, it is common to see Aloe Vera presented the following way on a label. Aloe Vera (**Aloe** Barbadensis)   I am somewhat okay with this, but many people we survey think that there are twice as many ingredients in the product because of the dual listing. The Skin Deep database does a marvelous job of helping out this problem because it offers both name forms on each ingredient they rank.

The message here is to research an ingredient you do not recognize.

Search the Databases: Feed Your Head

Your best resources for finding out product and chemical safety are really two very different databases. There are others that you can research as a consumer, but these two give you all the information you need and are written for lay people to understand.

Safe Cosmetics Skin Deep Database http://www.safecosmetics.org

National Institutes of Health Toxnet database.
http://toxnet.nlm.nih.gov/

Breaking them down:

Safe Cosmetics Skin Deep Database is what it says. This database ranks cosmetic and personal care products on a scale of 0 to 10 with 10 being unsafe. You can look for safe products based on their ranking system and you can drill into them deeper to see the ingredients concerns and comments down to the ingredient level. To be clear, the database is mostly about what is bad for you based on their compilation of a number of databases. Bad in this sense is only what a chemical will do to you from a perspective of toxicity, hormone disruption or some other malady that besets you. It does not deal with non-toxic reactions. For example, many people are allergic to the smell and contact from natural lavender oil. Synthetic lavender oil made by some companies contains phthalates which is a known hormone disrupter. On the database, natural lavender has a safe rating while synthetic a bad mark. This further begs the point that we have to understand what is good for us individually and what is not.

Toxnet is more complicated and does cover household products as well as a wide range of other products.

When you go on the Toxnet website, pick a simple common ingredient like SLS (Sodium Laureth Sulfate) and search it. Look at the precautions, safety issues and concerns as well as the function of the ingredient. Then try Methyl Paraben. This is another common ingredient in cosmetics and personal care. It is designed as a bactericide and will have different warnings. Toxnet is very much a scientists' and ingredient geek site that is simplified enough for the average mortal to understand. As you research Toxnet, it becomes more and more relevant and helpful. As your understanding and knowledge increases, Toxnet will help you make very solid decisions.

Google and Other Search Engines

Search engines are a wonderful source of ingredients, opinion and some facts. I use Google all the time to begin looking at trends balancing the many industry newsletters and blogs that flood me with the latest news, trends and product announcements.

How to use these search engines and what they offer is a very important process. Most of what I read on search engines is opinion. For example, four years ago while attending the Natural Products Expo West, this new wonder ingredient called Acai was being introduced on the supplier side of the convention where people like me go to look for ingredients. A year later at the expo, there were literally twenty companies with juices, candies and foods all containing Acai. Another year passed and there were only ten companies showing Acai and the web was full of pros and cons for the ingredient.

When using search engines, make sure that you separate fact from fiction and facts from opinion.

My recommendation for the best process is to research Skin Deep and Toxnet for the facts and go to Google for opinion and you connect the dots for yourself.

Wikipedia...Perhaps the Best of Search Engines

If you are not familiar with www.wikipedia.com, it is an online encyclopedia shared and contributed by anyone qualified to add a topic and expand on it. Wiki is a Hawaiian word that means quick. **Wikipedia** is a free, web based collaborative, multilingual encyclopedia project supported by the non-profit Wikimedia Foundation. Its 16 million articles (over 3.3 million in English) have been written collaboratively by volunteers around the world, and almost all of its articles can be edited by anyone with access to the site. Wikipedia was launched in 2001 and is currently the largest and most popular general reference work on the Internet. It is ranked 7th among all websites on a popularity basis.

So, take SLS and Methyl Paraben and look it up on Wikipedia. What you will see is that these chemicals are described based on their properties, reactions, purpose and history. What you will quickly see is a more scientific approach with some relevant opinion and sometimes conjectures.

Now, if you grab a product, look on the label and see a chemical or ingredient you do not know about or understand, you can go to Skin Deep to read what it says. Then go to Toxnet to find more details. From there, I recommend a quick look on Wikipedia and finally to Google for all the opinion and posturing.

All are valuable when held in context.

Creating Our Own Database

Toxicity is an interesting word. Like many words, it has a real meaning and a colloquial or everyday meaning. The way databases use toxicity as a word is the extreme definition of harm. Toxics everyday meaning is that a substance labeled with this word means that it is dangerous. Like most words, the meaning of toxic ranges from discomfort, to reaction and then finally to harmful.

Many things to me are toxic. Sometimes even some people because they are discomforting. So is true of things that I put in and on my body.

This topic is perhaps the most essential thing you can learn from this book and is also difficult to undertake.

Let's go back to the lavender oil example I use above. I am highly allergic to ragweed. I do not know if I am skin allergic to it, because I cannot get close enough to touch it. Lavender is a close cousin to ragweed. I not only sneeze uncontrollably, but I break out in itchy red stuff if I encounter natural lavender. Actually many people also have this malady and love the smell of synthetic lavender. Natural lavender is like poison ivy or oak to me. I am unaware of any human that is not allergic to poison ivy or oak, although I know dogs are immune. I know many people that are not allergic to lavender and some, like me that are highly allergic. The point? Lavender is a toxin to me!

Lavender is on Bob's (my) Toxic Database. Like many, I used to keep a mental record of what I was allergic to and what bothered me. When I started to create my own database in the form of a toxic journal, I started to see patterns emerge. For example, I have a similar yet lesser reaction to strawberries. The same is true of peach fuzz and yet I love to eat peaches if they are peeled. I love berries and most love me, but I have to be careful when I go out for a smoothie.

When I am in the mood for a smoothie, 95+% of the time I make them for myself. On those occasions when I see a smoothie store when I am out and about, I can't resist stopping. Some people have to have chocolate when they pass a chocolate store and I have to have smoothies.

I cannot just stop in any smoothie shop because most will not customize what they make. I also have a database of smoothie stores I can stop in and what they sell that I can have without reacting. So, I have to restrict what I can order at the Jamba Juice in Santa Monica, but when I am in Santa Barbara, I can satisfy any flavor urge because Blenders in the Grass will take things out or customize my smoothie the way I want it. Making sense?

Tolerances are also an important toxin to observe and put in your personal database. Again using me as an example, I realized at my ripe age that I have a gluten intolerance. Now that I learned this, I now understand why I did not want birthday cakes as a child.

Funny as it sounds, we as humans often need a defining moment to notice things. For some, a health scare breaks them free of their rigid maps that they have created for their lives. For some it is a simple 'ahha' moment of why they do not like something or react to it in such a way as to notice and register the reaction.

Creating and journaling the ingredients and foods that you react to unfavorably as well as favorably can and will go a long way to increasing your health and skin health.

To make the point, let's be silly for a moment. Say you go to a high-end skincare studio created by someone long since dead that was a self proclaimed expert. You walk in and tell them that you want to look younger. They sit you down, clean your face with their fruit acid cleanser, put some fruit acid exfoliant on your face and then put a "soothing" cream containing fruit acid in it on your face. They hand you a bag of samples and say try them for a week and come back.

All good business practices, but let's say you walk a block down the street and your face is on fire, red and very irritated. A reaction to fruit acid? Too much too fast? Sounds unusual, not really, it happened last year to Wendy and it literally took her a few days to calm her skin down.

In this case, we discovered that she had both a reaction to fruit acids and it was way too much.

The same thing happened to Wendy when she went to her medical esthetician right after her normal 6 month checkup at the dermatologist. The esthetician gave her some new makeup that was supposed to smooth and settle down her skin. Within an hour, she complained of burning and a dry itchy feel. Looking at the jar, there were no ingredients listed. What was easy for me to detect was a obviously high level of silica in the powdered product. I went to the website for the product and sure enough, the first ingredient was silica.

Again, in this case, Wendy's skin condition was allergic to the product and we suspect it was the silica. She now knows to look for silica in products before trying them. She also has a list of what not to buy.

Finally, on this point, creating your own list of no-no chemicals for you is important. Like that trend in the 1980's to get your "color palette" done by an expert to help you figure out what colors look best for your skin and hair color, so is this list of no-no ingredients.

Develop a List of Clean No-No's

MSG, Head & Shoulders, Dawn detergent, dryer sheets and laundry detergents. What do these toxins have in common? For me, these are products I once used but can no longer because I have built-down toxicity to them. Not built-up, but built-down!

I have a term for something I call Clean Intolerances called **Clean No-No's!** Simply what this means is things I used to eat or use, I can no longer use because I have cleaned up my act from both a diet and personal care perspective. These products have become intolerable for me because I now have a reaction to them. Once I was able to use these products, but now I react because I continually use my personal database to reduce and eliminate things I react to.

Innocent Overdose: How Products are made. Ingredient Subcomponents

This is a little more difficult to explain because we are all conditioned to believe that if there are ten ingredients on a label that we believe there are only ten. In the next bulleted item, I will cover a term called label content. This section deals with ingredients that often even the manufacturer does not know are in their products.

Say I have a lotion that is made up from five ingredients like avocado oil, vegetable glycerin and vegetable emulsifying wax along with a couple of other things. There are some things to consider that are important to me and should be important to you. Although this is nearly impossible for you to find out, the following should be a concern to manufacturers.

1. Is the ingredient whole and unprocessed?

2. If the ingredient is fabricated (like glycerin and most wax)... What is it made from to start? For example, wax can be petroleum based or vegetable based. If it is vegetable based, is it Palm oil or Coconut oil based. If it is palm based, is it from a sustainable manufacturer or one of the big palm oil companies stripping the rain forest?

3. Does the ingredient raw material manufacturer add stabilizer and germicides to protect the ingredient from contamination during transport?

4. Are the ingredients processed, irradiated or altered in any way?

Just as an example, say that a manufacturer uses one of those 'weasel phrases' like **No Parabens Added** to their label. When in good conscience, they know that each of their raw material ingredients is shipping in to them with parabens already added. There are already enough parabens in the raw materials so that they do not have to add any additional parabens.

Let me be clear that a label that says "No Parabens Added" is suspect, but I would sure rather see the label say No Parabens! Get the point?

Although the Certificate of Origin template does not require listing the sub ingredients, most of the people wanting to supply us now are presenting us a certificate of purity where they disclose any sub ingredients.

Also, although many manufacturers claim to be small and without resources, it is their responsibility to know what is in their ingredients and their finished products. Keys was once small and struggled to find ingredients that were whole and pure because we are founded by a sensitive skin Cancer recovering survivor.

An entire industry book could be written on this subject. The easiest suggestion for you is to find trusted advisors at your local apothecary or health food store and investigate manufacturers for their integrity.

Label Content:

Label content is a term that has no good side to it. The term means two things. Both are usually deceptive in intent.

1. It is acceptable by some manufacturers to not list an ingredient on the label if it is less than 1% of the total. Think this out a bit. If a company needs around 1.2% of a broad spectrum paraben, they might choose to use three parabens at less than 0.4% each so that it totals the targeted 1.2%.

2. Reverse label content is more sinister to me because you can include 0.0001% of an ingredient and actually list it on the label as some sort of benefit. What exactly does, "A Touch of Aloe" actually mean?

To explain this more is to simply say that it is not required that the manufacturer list an ingredient that is less than 1%. Most parabens and chemical enhancers only need be 0.5% to do their job. Therefore, they are not listed.

Second, a manufacturer can claim an effective ingredient like Aloe, Shea Butter or Acai even though there is not enough of the ingredient to have a positive effect.

Efficacy

Efficacy is different from label content in many ways and yet it can be used in a similar fashion. The simplest way I explain it is using the word amplitude. An ingredient that is effective is both the highest quality and in high enough proportion to do something for you.

This is about figuring out what works for you, what does not and why.

We are a pill society! Yep, have a problem take a pill. Have a disorder want a pill. Have a deficiency need a pill! The pills that we take fail or succeed on a term called efficacy. So is true and should be true of any products we use on our skin.

In a healthcare context, efficacy indicates the capacity for beneficial change or a therapeutic effect.

The concept of 'self-efficacy' is an important one in the self-management of chronic diseases because doctors and patients often do not follow best practice in using a treatment. For instance, a patient using a combined oral blood pressure pill to lower their BP may sometimes forget to take their pill at the prescribed time.

Boiling all these words down, does a product work for you or not! My definition of efficacy is individually based and not broad spectrum.

My efficacy definition: "Efficacy is the capacity to produce an effect on an individual basis."

Efficacy for skin health is based on the quality and quantity of an ingredient. As an example, I can buy an Aloe Vera that is cheap with low potency and use it is a very small percentage in a product. I can add some marketing phrase to the label like, "With the Coolness of Aloe" and people may believe they are getting a benefit when they are actually gaining nothing. To the contrary, I can search the world for the finest jet dried Aloe crystal and then use in high proportion. Then I might list on the label not only the ingredient, but how much is in the product as a percentage of the whole and the quality level of that Aloe.

Efficacy also defined is integrity of both purpose and effect on the individual.

Labels

The simplest thing I can say about labels is that they should be simple!

Jack Welch, of General Electric, was a sort of icon and mentor to me in my corporate life as a CEO. His pragmatic, take no prisoners approach made my life a lot simpler. His quote, "That only self-confident people can be simple," stuck with me most of my career. I liked it because most of the time, I found people operating on the 'complexity breeds complexity strategy'. The more complex, the safer I am in my job.

When I joined the natural products industry, I found the opposite seemed to be the rule. Complex formulas made from complex things were more the norm. Companies accused the big guys of trying to make things too complex. No one could agree on what to put on a label and how. The answer seemed to be to start some group, association or club that would study, recommend or define everything. I saw this like trying to design an elephant by committee. Futile at best and we already know what an elephant looks like.

I sat for an entire day in a meeting where chemists debated what the term "Natural "means. Only to relegate the job to a committee that meets twice a year.

Some say that we should have the Latin names on the label to make labels more 'clear' to consumers of what is in the products they buy.

Latin Clear? What percentage of the general population speaks Latin? We did an intercept study at the industry's largest tradeshow in Anaheim California a few years back. We asked these industry experts attending the Natural Products Expo West show what ten ingredients were based on their INCI names. Not one got all ten correct. These were industry experts, chemists from big companies. I thought, how do you expect consumers to know what an ingredient is if industry people do not know. And worse, how do I translate Latin into French so that I can sell in Canada and the EU....Okay, just kidding! I seem to get these activist moments.

So rather than trying to sit in a committee and try to figure out what consumers should see on a label, we did the unthinkable. We went to the streets and asked them. Not in some sort of navigated constructed focus group, we just asked them.

Here is what they said:

- I want to know what the product does.
- I want to know it does what it says.
- I want to know what is in it (ingredients) in plain English.
- When you put something in a product that is supposed to do something, I want to know how much of it you put in there.
- I want to know are the ingredients good high quality or cheap versions.
- I don't have time for marketing speak, so please just tell me what to expect.

The list goes on and on, but I think you get the drift. Over stated, what we have heard from every corner of this country is that people want simple. Simple products that do what they say. People do not want their time wasted.

So rather than sitting in a committee debating what we think is right, we chose to redesign our labels three years ago to match what the customers are asking for. We are not claiming that it is right or wrong, just responsiveness to our customers. Over the last three years, we have continued to change our labels to make them simpler and easier to interpret. Still waiting for that industry committee, we continue to modify and migrate to more information in its simplest form.

Hiding in the GRAS (Not a typo)

There is a term in the industry that you should be aware of called GRAS. This is an acronym for **G**enerally **R**ecognized **A**s **S**afe. What this term means is that a chemical has been used long enough that the industry believes that it is safe and does not warrant further testing. As we go through the products on the market, I have come to recognize that GRAS really means generally recognized as okay because we did not hurt anyone so far. GRAS is a term that does not take into regard hormonal disruption, birth defects or long-term disorders. What it really means is that the GRAS ingredients do not send you to the hospital right away. I can say this without sounding like an activist because there is and has been no long range testing of 99% of the ingredients used in personal care or household products. What it generally means is that a GRAS ingredient is safe until proven that it is not. Sort of sounds like CYA (Cover Your Ass) to me for chemists. It is a catchall term that I dislike and I find some of the larger "natural" brands are using the term a little too much.

Fragrance and Unscented

It is nearly impossible to make a natural product without scent or any smell. There are some that are close, but I am concerned that being low scent also means they are less effective.

Most of the exotic French fragrance houses produce some marvelous products. They are as close to natural as humanly possible and usually are made from hundreds of ingredients. Sorry to say, these are not the ones used in the lotion that sells for $4.95 in the big box stores.

Fragrances used in personal care products are cheap very powerful chemical concoctions. I was in a meeting and someone said that Tide laundry detergents fragrance has over 100 chemicals to make it unique. The same person told me that most of all the laundry powders the company produces are all the same product, but with a different fragrance.

Most synthetic fragrances that I have seen contain phthalates to make them longer lasting. Phthalates are hormone disrupters that are banned in the EU and in California. It is also very important to understand that most companies that mark their products with the term 'fragrance' do not mean it has one ingredient. More than likely that fragrance is 30, 40 or 50 chemicals! Based on industry standards, fragrance is considered one ingredient and often is not listed because the 'fragrance' is so powerful that the product only needs a fraction of 1% to achieve the desired scent.

Most unscented products use a contra-chemical to mask the smell. There is a common belief, that "No Tears" baby shampoos actually have an anesthetic in them. They still can irritate and turn the eyes red, but it does not burn. I do not know if this is an urban myth or true. What I do know is that there are companies whose entire purpose is to develop a masking contra-chemical to make unscented products.

Basically, the way it works is that I could develop a product with twenty ingredients that smells like an old spare tire fresh off the rim. I would send this completed formula to one of these companies and they would make a chemical that would mask the smell and make it virtually scent free. More chemicals? Yes! Phthalates? Most likely!

Here are a couple of truisms:

1. Any scent that lasts more than 10 minutes and is floral is probably synthetic and most likely contains phthalates unless it is marked phthalate free.

2. Unscented products use a contra-chemical that cannot be detected by smelling with the nose. As a trick, when you smell a product marked unscented or scent-free, don't smell it with your nose. Smell it with your mouth. Yep, open your mouth and breathe in. Those tastes you are experiencing are the chemicals.

3. Fragrance is not one ingredient. If it is synthetic it is a large number of component chemicals.

Government Controls

The simplest way to tell you about the control of cosmetics and personal care in the United States is that there isn't any! Yep, the industry is self-policing. Enough said?

Chapter Tools

1. Chemicals can be bad for you personally as well as because you are human. Meaning that what is bad for you as a species is obvious. What is bad for you individually is not as easy to figure out.

2. Research all of your products against the www.safecosmetics.org Skin Deep database.

3. Lineup all your personal care products and cosmetics and look at the ingredients to see which are unsafe according to Skin Deep.

4. Review all your products for their rating on the database.

5. Put all the products ranked as unsafe on your dining room table and take a picture of them all before you return them to the manufacturer.

6. Create your own personal database with the following fields:
   a. Reaction Toxins
   b. Intolerance Toxins
   c. Clean No No's

7. If there are no ingredients on the label do not buy the product.

8. If you cannot pronounce or don't recognize and ingredient, research what it is before you buy it.

As an additional note, I have listed various resources in the back of the book.

Chapter 7: Safe Cosmetics...There are none!

I am sorry to say, there are no safe cosmetics that I have found for one reason of the other. I must quickly add that there are safer alternative and some cosmetics that are downright nasty.

Universally, when I am in front of customers, doctors, estheticians, makeup artists, actors and cosmeticians, the question is always the same. "When is Keys going to create a makeup line?" My answer is when I can find safe ingredients that have the right colors and staying power.

This is a tough chapter for me because it flies in the face of just about every conventional thinker in the makeup industry. My thinking is simple and controversial because I believe that the New Cosmetics is a combination of clear beautiful skin and transparent color that creates an allure. I believe that this is for both men and women where both choose the intensity and combination of colors without cover-up.

As a note, in preparing for this chapter I spent some time with product based makeup artists from companies that sell in very high end department stores. These people actually work for the brand and rent space inside the stores. Universally I am pleased to say that all of these people are conscious of the trend toward natural makeup and skin care. When I addressed the issue head on, they had answers that were not some company party line. These individuals know what they are talking about and are pretty sharp when it comes to skin.

Ironically, as I began to study their ingredients, they were not too bad for some of the brands and I began to recognize that it was the drug store low end brands that seem to be of the greatest concern in my research. Like the marvelous French perfume houses that create naturally derived fragrance, the high end cosmetics use many of the same ingredients that I use in our products. Unfortunately almost all cosmetics have parabens as a preservative. Pretty good overall.

As I began to look at the "natural" cosmetics, overall they were also good, but used some questionable ingredients that have an even higher concern level to me.

For example, I found the use of silica and mica as well as iron oxide being used in natural products under the moniker of "Mineral Makeup."

For example, silica is used to make glass and computer chips. It is considered perfectly safe except when it is in a powdered form. Inhaling finely divided crystalline silica dust in very small quantities over time can lead to silicosis, bronchitis, or cancer, as the dust becomes lodged in the lungs and continuously irritates them, reducing lung capacities. Silica does not dissolve over time. This effect can be an occupational hazard for people working with sandblasting equipment, products that contain powdered crystalline silica and so on. Children, asthmatics of any age, allergy sufferers, and the elderly can be affected with higher reaction levels.

In respects other than inhalation, pure silicon dioxide is inert and harmless. Clean silicon dioxide yields no fumes and is insoluble in the body.

So here is the rub. As manufacturers perfect mineral makeup, they are creating smaller and smaller dust like versions of silica. Putting these into a powder that you dust your face with begins to create the possibility and maybe probability that could harm people over time.

The situation is less than humorous when you find that government bodies like OSHA and the EPA require people that work around silica to wear respirators. Yes, there is no regulatory body looking at the safety of makeup.

When I started the book, I fully intended to differentiate 'good' and 'bad' makeup. What I ultimately found is that natural and high-end store brands are much better from a chemical and ingredient perspective than cheaper drug store brands. The problem is that as I studied more and listened to reactions of people, I found that all makeup is flawed in some way or the other.

My belief came from a combination of studying the communications of the skin and the concern I have studying the chemicals in cosmetics. Later in this chapter, I will talk about my concept for 'Clear Cosmetics' and how it was some friends in the TV and motion picture industry that brought this clarity.

Everything in moderation! Bare it all when you can.

Before I jump into my concept for clear cosmetics, I want to touch on one last point about makeup. Let's just say that I did not convince you to go into public with nothing on but your smile! Then what I want you to try for me is to bare it all as often as you can. For example, remember from the Skin 101 chapter that the skin breathes, absorbs and expels both gases and liquid. For your skin health, let your skin breath as often as possible. Despite what you have been told, try my mini-regime as often as you can for a month. So, here it goes.

- At night wash your face with a mild natural soap that is slightly alkaline and go to bed.
- As often as you can, wake in the morning and wash with the same natural soap. Do not put anything on your skin for as long as possible...that means no foundation or makeup. If you can avoid color around the eyes, cheek and lips it would be great.
- Use a natural moisturizer instead of a foundation and put color on your eyes, lips and cheeks.
- Wear a big hat and/or sunblock that is broad spectrum when out in the world. Remembering that UVA is the aging rays and that they penetrate car windows as well as most office windows, make sure what you use is broad spectrum. When you get home, wash it off with your natural cleanser.
- Do not use any products on your face with alcohol in them during the trial period. If you use an herbal toner, make sure it does not contain natural lavender oil.

Again, try this for a month as often as possible. Then add your daily moisturizer back in. Notice the changes. Also, listen carefully when your friends notice the change. Do not be surprised that they say you look happier. This is because I believe the 'real you' is now shining through.

The following is an article I wrote for our blog. Although this plugs our products in the creation of a regime, you can select and use the products you wish.

Clear Cosmetics – Keys Makeup

I told you earlier that when I am in front of customers, doctors, estheticians, makeup artists, actors and cosmeticians, the question is always the same. "When is Keys going to create a makeup line?" My answer is when I can find safe ingredients that have the right colors and staying power.

I began looking at traditional makeup about four years ago. I studied conventional makeup products as well as the mineral makeup. What I found in common was a group of minerals and compounds that are earth derived mostly from oxides and rock ground into small particles These minerals are then suspended either in a cream, lotion or dry compressed.

Upon further investigation, I found that many lipsticks (most), colorants like eye shadow and tints all contained lead, mica, silica, iron oxide and even some minerals that have low dose radiation. When I discovered this, I wondered why the companies producing makeup did not use berries, extracts, plant parts and other safer ingredients. As I studied further, I realized that using the "more natural" ingredients did not work nearly as effectively as their mineral alternatives. Why? The answer is that most, if not all, non-mineral colors are weak and have low staying power. Mostly because most mineral based makeup are opaque in nature where fruit based colorants are more transparent and are water-soluble.

I have continued to study over the years and check in with friends in the industry in a collaborative effort. In fact, at the last Natural Products Expo West, friends in the industry scoured the show looking for natural colorant ingredients. My friend Kathleen Beaton would ring my cell phone and tell me of a booth she had found that had something that looked good. As a premier makeup artist, I respected her eye for color and she respected my scientific ability to very quickly determine whether the particular ingredient was clean, green and had the staying power. That day was spent running back in forth a few steps behind Kathleen. Then the phone would ring and it would be someone else looking for something and wondering if I had seen it. At the same show, we checked in with the makeup companies and the ones new to offering makeup. Still the same old same old minerals.

Los Angeles – Makeup's Center of the Universe

As a man, I appreciate makeup, but cannot totally understand it. Checking in with the idea of creating a makeup line on occasion, I did not really understand a lot until recently when I was in LA. We were scheduled for a big Hollywood local event. Being an LA boy, I took advantage of the event to arrive early and leave town late. I had lunch with Kathleen Beaton one day in Venice Beach, checked in with Ele Keats who is my favorite actor and was on the set of Weeds staring at the beautiful skin of Mary Louise Parker. With the help of all, I finally got it! There is the color and there is the canvas! Probably obvious to most women, I realized that the majority of makeup is to smooth out and even out the complexion, so color can be layered on. What I realized is that makeup is like painting a portrait in reverse. To start, an artist takes white paint and covers the canvas with several coats to smooth out and make the finish consistent. Then they layer color on the white canvas to create the image they want. Layer after layer, they build up color for the final image. Makeup has traditionally been the same. Take foundations and minerals to the face to create a smooth even finish. Then add color to finish.

Kathleen calls her art "painting faces." For years now, we get together and talk about her efforts to create a makeup line. As my friend, I struggled to help her, but it was difficult because I did not get it. I respect Kathleen's work and her abilities. She is a great makeup artist and has one of the toughest jobs in LA because she often does makeup for TV commercials using everyday people as the stars of the commercials. Now with high definition, it is even tougher. When I see those commercials, I cannot believe how natural looking those people look.

The Hollywood event came. Standing next to the stage listening to Ed Begley talk, I was suddenly in the embrace of this gorgeous woman. Ele Keats had surprised me with a visit down from the Hollywood Hills. She looked radiant and her skin just glowed. I know that she is a devout fan of Solar Rx and Luminos. It was a weekend and LA always turns out in their finest designer grunge. Still, in this sea of beautiful people Ele just glowed. Her skin was clear, even, natural and with a dewy glow. Like always, she looked perfect and the infectious smile of Ele Keats topped of her look.

From LA, I headed to Portland Oregon for the opening of the new Fez Studio. I love Portland because it is a cool city with lots to do and see. Most of the year Portland is wet and rainy. One of the first things you notice is that people have gorgeous clear skin. No sun damage here! Talking with mostly women at the event, I could not help but notice that they had little to no foundation with color only on the lips, eyes and maybe cheeks. It all became clear to me in a flash! I was already in the makeup business and the reason that Fez Studio and the many natural makeup stores that carry our products was because what we were able to do to get the natural look. It was because we make Clear Cosmetics.

Clear Cosmetics Is Keys Makeup

How can there be such a thing as Clear Cosmetics? Remember what I said that painting of the canvas to prime it before the artist can start. The purpose of that and a concealing foundation on the face is to create a smooth even look before adding color. Personally, I think there is nothing prettier than the glow of naturally healthy skin. As I thought about Ele and Mary Louise, I realized that their natural glowing dewy skin was incredibly sexy because the real person shows through.

I realized I was in the cosmetic business because I created products that offer two primary things for the skin. The secret of clear cosmetics is that using our regime, the skin heals and gets a natural even glow. Our light diffraction technology using natural Aloe crystals further smoothes the appearance of the skin diffusing light to create a glowing beautiful energy for women and men of all ages.

Painting Faces: Luminos Background – How it began!

Keys were thrust into the Hollywood scene with our Eye Butter. Invited to present Eye Butter to 300 Hollywood makeup artists I was exposed to a lot of industry jargon. What struck me the most was that the makeup artists referred to themselves as "face painters."

As Eye Butter grew in popularity, I realized that we had something different. Eye Butter was different than anything else because it softened, illuminated and brightened the eyes. Makeup artist liked it because they kept telling me that it is like using a clear foundation that hides defects without covering them up. They also liked that my products grab the makeup so that it goes on thinner and smoother.

I really did not take notice of what they said or why Eye Butter was so interesting until a makeup artist asked me to create a new product for a new TV show.

The challenge was to create a moisturizer foundation that would create a soft focus filter for the skin. They wanted a moisturizer that would scatter light to trick the camera and permit the same makeup to be used indoors and outdoors without needing to change for each lighting situation.

The reason this makeup artist asked me to create this new product was that she noticed that Eye Butter did what she wanted. She started to use Eye Butter all over the face. Her request, do what I did in Eye Butter in a moisturizer form.

My career began in optical physics at a Polaroid Research & Development company. Photographic and printing technology is either an additive or a subtractive color. The best and smoothest color uses subtractive color components. Today the best photo printers use subtractive technology. It is why your digital camera pictures look so clean, crisp and vivid.

Makeup has been the same since cave dwellers painted their faces. Solid additive color rubbed, brushed and placed strategically on the face. Same then as it is now!

What I realized in designing Luminos is that I had shifted from the world of additive to subtractive technology.

What does Luminos do and how does it work?

If you have read anything I have written, you already know I am a geek. I believe that when you understand why a product works, you know how to better utilize it. So is true of Luminos!

The technology is revolutionary to the world of makeup. It has been around in the world of photography since the late 1800's. It is the world of diffraction, diffusion and subtractive color.

Let's start with the challenge.

Create a moisturizer that creates a soft focus filter for the skin...not the camera!

The world of high definition photography, television and motion pictures has made critical and revealing the skin of actors, newscasters and everyday people shot in "high-def." The solution for most news broadcasts has been to pull those cameras back to show space above and below the newscasters' body. Those old torso shots are now full length.

Since the beginning of motion pictures and then TV, the solution was to put a filter on the camera to soften the look. In the world of High Def, everything has to be sharp and crisp. High Def cameras are often four times as sharp, crisp and revealing as old film and television. The early solution was to use more and more makeup. As motion pictures and television tried to make the actors look more natural and less phony, conventional makeup did just the opposite. In addition, as the green movement took over Hollywood, that dead dry mineral makeup look was changed out to a youthful glow.

The natural look is in and age is no longer an excuse. Young actors with outstanding skin like Rachel McAdams do not want to hide it. Now in her 40's Mary Louise Parker has gorgeous skin and does not want to hide it. Using any form of opaque makeup covers and hides...and everyone knows it. It has become a huge challenge for the professional makeup artist.

Analyzing what I had created with Eye Butter is not a cover-up, but a new direction in makeup called refraction.

How Eye Butter works and now Luminos is that it does not cover up, but diffuses the light in such a way as to trick not only the camera, but also the eye. To understand, you must understand the difference between traditional makeup and where we are going with our new field of Clear Cosmetics. Now, rather than an opaque multilayer foundation made from minerals and then layering color, we propose that the new look is a Keys diffraction foundation, adding spot color to enhance. Instead of hiding the skin using layers of thick base, with Luminos the skin glows evenly and softens the skin without a filter on the camera. Luminos is truly like a soft focus filter for the skin!

Happiness is the best cosmetic

A smile is contagious, laughter makes you young and why brides glow…..

Chapter 8: Safer Personal Care Products...a challenge!

Keys is really in the **'person care'** business. Not the personal care business! Maybe someday we will be in the cosmetics business, but not as I write this book. Technically, we are a natural skincare product company that focuses on people with sensitive skin. We were thrust into the Hollywood scene with the challenge of making a natural product that performed better than conventional products.

Our customers are mostly people with sensitive skin and most use our products, not because they are chemical-free, but because what is makes their skin look like.

Once I was told by a green advocate actor that she really wants a product that is safe and makes her look good. She quickly told me that she makes a living with her face and if products do not perform, she will not use them.

All of this said, when I started my study of the skin care and personal care sector I expected it to be somewhat equal to makeup. I was wrong. Personal care is perhaps the most volatile and scariest product group when it comes to skin health and skin safety.

I started my research on the Skin Deep report looking at the worst ranked products. I studied the ingredients, the types of ingredients and the sheer number used in each product. I was amazed, but blown away when I went into the anti-aging sector of the personal care industry. Not only were there many questionable ingredients, but the amount of chemicals in some products astounded me.

I read somewhere that the average ingredients in personal care products was around 35 chemicals compounds. When I began to research the anti-aging market sector I found products with over 50 compounds were more the norm than the exception. Many of these products compounds were totally unknown to me and were considered exclusive ingredients that are proprietary to their designers. Then I thought maybe these single ingredients on a label may have 20, 30 or 40 sub-ingredient components. It frankly made my head hurt.

Again, I found that the natural products were by far the simplest and mostly used whole oils, butters and essential oil. Again, the high-end department stores were not terrible. My complaint about them is still about the parabens, but they used some fine ingredients warranting their higher prices due to their higher cost loads to manufacture.

It is the middle of the road, drug store and big box brands that seem to be chemically out of control. One shampoo I found had three forms of sulfates, three forms of parabens, four forms of glycols and two forms of silicone in one product.

My hope for both this chapter and the one on cosmetics is that I would be able to make recommendations of brands and trends. I am sorry to say that these both have become somewhat minor chapters with me offering my perspective of potential alternative thinking.

I truly believe that the healthiest skin is clean uncovered skin. I believe that some chemicals used in skin care and personal care products is harmful both long and short term.

Next time you are in a drug store or the personal care aisle in a big box retailer, spend a few moments reading the label ingredients. Don't worry what they are or what they do, just count the number. As a note, bring a magnifying glass because you will probably need it.

As a parting comment, I walked into a Vitamin Shoppe store where I buy some of my supplements. There was a sunscreen in a floor display that had a big "All Natural" headline. I looked at the product, flipped it over as I usually do and searched for the ingredient deck. All I saw was an active ingredient list containing Oxybenzone. I thought all natural? No way! As I started to put the product back, I felt the label move and I was curious. I picked at the edge of the label and it slid open like a label that you see on an insecticide at the hardware store. When I opened the label, the complete ingredient deck was there. The only thing that looked natural to me was the water. There were at least 40 chemicals in this product and it confirmed my fear that the personal care sector is the scariest of all. Especially in the midrange price point market.

Keys Clear Cosmetics Regime and the Keys Challenge

First, the regime I want you to try is the price of one item at a Nordstrom brand makeup counter. All of the items combined are less than some lipsticks at Barney's in LA. So try it, but please be religious about it for ten days.

There are four products in the regime or maybe even only three.

Here are the products:

1. Island Rx Foaming Wash

2. Luminos Moisturizer Clear Foundation

3. Eye Butter Clear Eye Enhancer

4. Solar Rx Moisturizing Sunblock

Island Rx Foaming Wash

Island Rx Foaming Wash is a cleanser adjusted to be slightly alkaline to clean and tone the skin. The simple formulation contains no chemicals that cause inflammation of the skin and the Clary Sage actually reduces inflammation. After turning jojoba, avocado and olive oil into a cleanser using an ancient process, we add back in avocado oil, Clary sage essential oil and blood orange essential oil. These oils also serve specific purposes that clean, hydrate, condition and exfoliate the skin without using harsh scrubs, toners or chemical peels.

Luminos

Luminos was developed for Hollywood to create a glowing illusion to improve the look of the skin under high definition photography and motion pictures. What we later discovered was that Luminos also created that look for everyday use as a clear makeup. Luminos contains pharmaceutical grade ingredients in high proportions combined with a concentration of Aloe Vera crystals that act as millions of little prisms on the skin. It naturally smoothes the finish of the skin while providing a glow that increases the depth and definition of the skin cells. Applied lightly over a freshly cleaned face with Island Rx also provides a natural barrier from pollutant, hydrocarbons and allergens that affect the look and condition of the skin.

Eye Butter

Eye Butter starts with a very special cucumber extract that assures that the long chain polysaccharides are intact offering firming and fine line reduction around the eyes. Wild crafted grade Shea butter from Ghana is blended to soothe the eye tissue as well as plumping the tissue to give a fuller look. We then add our Aloe Crystals to create the same illusion as Luminos, but for the eyes. Eye Butter melts at skin temperature and is quickly absorbed leaving a slight tack to grab makeup as it is lightly brushed around the eyes. In a few minutes, it sets to hold the makeup.

Solar Rx

Our Solar Rx is a moisturizing sunblock designed for everyday use. It is very similar to Luminos with the addition of uncoated zinc oxide. The zinc oxide provides protection for UVA and UVB radiation while also acting as a natural anti-inflammatory reducing skin redness. Remember some of our other articles quoting the Skin Cancer Foundation that 90% of all visible skin aging is from UVA and UVB radiation. Solar Rx prevents increased exposure while also reconditioning the skin and repairing sun damage.

How To Use the Regimes:

In the morning, wash your face with Island Rx foaming wash applying the foam to wet skin using your fingers to cleanse the skin and lightly exfoliate the skin. Then apply Solar Rx evenly and lightly to the face, neck and backs of your hands. Then take your ring finger to apply an ample amount of Eye Butter letting your finger warm it for a few moments. Lightly pat the Eye Butter around the eye below and on the lid. Make sure it is smooth. (note: many people also put Eye Butter on their lips before they use lipstick to soften and moisturize the lips). Now apply makeup as desired around the eyes, cheeks and the lips. Do not use any foundation, but if you must, do it lightly.

At night, repeat the above process replacing Solar Rx with Luminos.

Now for the challenge…there always has to be a challenge, right?

Follow Wendy's Regime for ten days. If you want, shoot a before and after picture. Notice the difference in your skin! More importantly, listen carefully to your friends and family to see when they notice the changes in you.

Lastly, follow Ele Keats best beauty secret. Smile!

Chapter 9: Green Washing:

As consumers, chemicals in products are really all of our fault?

My Time to Rant!

Have you noticed how many "natural products" appeared on the market so quickly. It was just a year ago that many of these companies, now with natural products, were disputing the safety concerns of some of the chemicals they use. Now, you cannot open a magazine or turn on a TV or Google without seeing an ad for a brand that used to be anything but natural. Now they are saying we are paraben free or No SLS or no glycols....excuse me I got that wrong, they are saying no parabens added and no glycols added and Sodium Laureth Sulfate free.

Green Washing defined: Jumping on the natural bandwagon in the advertising and branding with much the same product as the non-green version and in some cases the same product.

We used to have a phrase/idiom in high tech we used when a competitor jumped ahead of us with a new product. The half joke and half-truth was our phrase, "The product will be available in 6 months and literature is available in volume shipments today."

I am all for products getting greener and cleaner. I want to support these companies and encourage them to join us at the Campaign for Safe Cosmetics (www.safecosmetics.org). The facts remain that the natural sector of the skin care, cosmetics and household products sector is outgrowing the conventional and these companies want not to lose anything. So, hopefully it will be true that the products will follow.

'Free and Clear' as we discovered does not mean chemical-free. Opponents claim everything is a chemical.

Do chemists really add and engineers subtract? All this is very confusing even as an industry insider.

It seems the model is to lead with the marketing and figure out if they have to follow with products. Slap a green label on that white bottle that you cannot see through, put a new label on it and using the words 'Free, Clear, Green and All-Natural' on the label does not mean it is safe.

One supplier alluded to me that they were asked to add parabens to their ingredient at higher levels as to assure that the total paraben level of a final product was enough to make sure that bacteria would not grow. Hmm, I thought, that is what 'no parabens added' means. In a sort of insidious way, the manufacturer used another term we coined in high tech: Weasel Words! Because they list an ingredient as PEG 150 and it happens to contain enough parabens to protect the product, they only have to list the PEG on the label....I.e. no parabens added!

Let me give you a personal example of what I am talking about here.

When we created our original Eye Butter, we used cucumber extract that was made from organic cucumber, skinned, seeded and then juiced and filtered. We prototyped our Eye Butter with the pure juice for testing purposes. We knew that we were going to have to buy the juice from somewhere or make it ourselves. We quickly realized that we could not find a supplier of natural juices designed for the cosmetics and personal care industry. So, we started making our own and distilling it to reduce microbiology issues.

About two years into the project I agreed to attend a meeting with a salesperson from a company claiming to have natural cucumber juice that was filtered, but not refined. You can only imagine my excitement and I agreed to the meeting.

I showed up and met the salesperson. He handed me the sample. I opened it and smelled it. It smelled like cucumber and it was clear in color the way I expected it to be. What happened next was shocking to the salesperson. What happened next was an interesting study in body language...the salesperson's that is.

What I did was take a swig of the liquid. After all, if it was natural there would be no problem. The salesperson visibly twitched and started to say, "Are you Crazy." Only the Are You came out before he caught himself.

It tasted terrible and before the salesperson could speak, I was headed out of the room toward the lab and our spectral chromatograph. The tests? Three types of parabens at twice the level expected. Looking at the Certificate of Origin sheet that accompanied the sample? No mention of anything but cucumber. Later, I found out from one of our engineers that the COA must only explain the main ingredients origin.

This left a bad taste in my mouth both literally and figuratively.

Unfortunately, this story is more the norm than the exception!

What also happens is that a company will substitute one ingredient for another. Say a company used SLS in their products, but the uproar caused them to change that ingredient out so that they could claim it had no SLS. All the time knowing that the new chemical was identical to SLS but with a different name.

A bigger problem to me are the many terms created by advertising agencies or marketing people. You know, Weasel Words!

So here is a list of Weasel Words that I jotted down after a trip to a grocery store near where I was staying.

Green Washing Weasel Words:

1. Free and Clear
2. Earth Derived
3. Green
4. Made from Plants
5. natural (small n)
6. Original Scent
7. No Parabens Added
8. No SLS (while having four other sulfates on the label)

The other deceptions are pictures of flowers on the bottle, little kids smiling or even a bunny while the back of the label has more bullets and no ingredients. There is usually also a big section on what to do if you get the product on your skin or in your eyes. One of the products I looked at had a number of seals on the back from organizations that they sponsor. You know the seals that you send money and you get to use the seal. And what difference should it make that the Sierra Club seal is on the back of a toilet bowl cleaner. The bottle has a green dispenser cap. That should mean something, right!

Now we use those words, Chemical-Free, No SLS, No Parabens, No Glycols, Gluten-Free. That is because we are free of synthetic chemicals, we do not use parabens or allow them in our raw materials. We test to make sure that we have no glycols and we are gluten-free because we do not use any gluten in our products. The difference between weasel words and marketing terms? Integrity!

All of us are really at fault because we constantly ask for more for less.

Yes, we as consumers are the reason all these chemicals exist in our products. In defense of the hard working chemists in all those big companies, they did not add chemicals to add them. For the exact same reason as they are now switching to "greener" ingredients is the strong marketing trend that is pushing the natural cosmetics, skincare and household products business. Just like the last 60 years, marketers evolve their products based on consumer trends.

Since the 1950's, television and Madison Avenue advertising executives came on the scene, the process of developing new trends and new directions for products is based on a need for product differentiation. Back in Silicon Valley, to describe differentiation, we even used the term, "Whiter Brighter" for our hard disks. Meaning what are the feature and benefits of the product. That whiter brighter term came from laundry detergents ads and stuck in high tech as industry jargon. The irony to me was that I jumped from an industry using the metaphoric term to one where it is an everyday term.

So, what has happened over time is that a product is often conceived in the marketing office. Then it is fleshed out at the advertising agency and then the chemist is asked to perform the miracle.

To make the point, I was looking at a product for reducing and eliminating wrinkles. There were over 50 ingredients listed in 1 point type. Binocular magnifiers on my head, I began to read the ingredients. Some were familiar ingredients because I use them. Some botanicals, fruit oils and some vegetable ingredients. I knew most of them and what they did, but what snapped for me was this trend I was seeing that related to trends from the 1950's and why they were used.

We affectionately often say Chemists Add and Engineers Subtract in our company because each year we see the average number of ingredients in personal care products and household products keep going up and up.

What I saw though in this one product was my life flashing before my eyes watching TV commercials while I growing up.

What I realized is that we as consumers asked for something and the chemist obliged by adding more and more chemicals. It is simply just a part of the marketing loop.

Consumers Ask - Marketing Listen - Chemists React –

New Product is born.

Here is what I mean.

Follow me as a consumer asking a chemist for things compressed down over 25 years:

- *Consumer:* My Ivory Soap won't suds in my hard water! *Chemist:* We can exchange the soap flakes for Sodium Laureth Sulfate, it is sudsy in all types of water!
- *Consumer:* My lotion is runny in the summer and too thick in the winter! *Chemist:* No problem, we can add glycols to make it consistent.
- *Consumer:* I want a bigger bottle! *Chemist:* No problem, we can put this chemical called Methyl Paraben in it and it won't grow bacteria for ten years.
- *Consumer:* I want my lotion to be scent free! *Chemist:* Hmmm can't do that, but the chemists have invented a masking fragrance that can counter the smell!
- *Consumer:* I am tired of getting shampoo in my baby's eyes and they cry because it burns. *Chemist:* No problem, we can add a numbing agent to the shampoo so it won't burn.
- *Consumer:* I want my house to smell like lavender all day. *Chemist:* You bet, we will just add Phthalates to the synthetic fragrance and it will last longer.
- *Consumer:* I want my cheese to not spoil so quickly! *Chemist:* Sure, we will just put some of that Triclosan biocide in the plastic packaging. *Consumer:* Won't that hurt me? *Chemist:* Don't think so, but we have not tested it!
- *Consumer:* I want my colored fabrics to look brighter! *Chemist:* Sure thing, we will put some phosphorus in your SLS based

detergent. *Consumer:* Will that hurt me? *Chemist:* No, but you will glow under blacklight!

- *Consumer:* I don't want my lipstick to kiss off.....
- *Consumer:* I want to smell different than others using the same cologne....
- *Consumer:* I want my hair color to look naturally blonde even though I am a redhead....

I think you get the picture. We ask and they respond because it differentiates their products from the competition and they sell more.

Now we have a whole new generation of consumers that want natural products. They want to look like they have no makeup on, but still look young. Our aging society wants to stay young while still living the same lifestyle that caused us to look old. A tall order and chemists are doing their best to accommodate. But for those that do not understand green chemistry or having to "cook" something versus tossing chemicals together, it is tough and breaking the best of them.

I don't know if this is true, but I was told by an industry person that the average personal care product today, in our sector, has 38 chemicals in them. Keys products average eight ingredients and have claimed functionality...meaning they do something. So, I went to the Safe Cosmetics database and sure enough, almost all of the natural products ranged from around 5 to 11 ingredients. A quick guess and I would have to say the average is about the same as ours...about eight!

I could go on and on.

Chapter Tools

1. If the ingredients are not listed on a product label do not buy it!
2. If you cannot pronounce an ingredient name, find out what it is and how it is made. The safe bet is don't buy it.
3. Get a list of the Marin County Cancer Project/Search for the Cause Dirty 30 chemicals list and go through your home. Return the products to the store you bought it from and tell them that you want to return the product because it has a Dirty 30 chemical in it. (This list is available from www.teensturninggreen.com or the Keys website)
4. Take the Dirty 30 list to your store to help you read labels before buying products.
5. Shop in the natural section of your super market or better yet, buy from a local natural food store that has trusted advisors and who care about what goes on your body.
6. Become an advocate by supporting the Safe Cosmetics Act in Congress.
7. Subscribe to the Safe Cosmetics blog and learn (www.safecosmetics.org)

Chapter 9: Anti-Aging, the Secret is Not in a Bottle

OK, set the book down and hold out your forearms. One up and one down. Notice a difference? If no, you protect your skin from UV damage and this is your biggest anti-aging secret. Notice a difference? Spots, dark patches, wrinkles, scales, warts, moles etc. UVA damage. Yep, the number one anti-aging secret is UV avoidance.

90% of all visible skin aging comes from Ultra Violet (UV) radiation. Yep, 90%! This is not a made up number, but listed by the National Institutes of Health.

Our star, the sun, provides life giving heat and balance. It also produces a wide array of radiation that strikes the earth. Our atmosphere blocks and/or filters out various forms of radiation.

UV radiation comes in three currently cataloged forms. UVA, UVB and UVC radiation. UVA, we call the UV Aging rays. UVB the UV Burning rays and UVC the UV Cancer rays. Fortunately our earth filters out most of the UVC and UVA rays. UVC is very rare to find hitting the earth and UVA is less in amplitude as UVB rays.

To put it in perspective, at one end of the visible spectrum are the red wavelengths. Just next to them is the infrared spectrum that we feel in the form of radiated heat. Toward the blue end of the spectrum are the UVA radiation bands followed closely by what is called "Soft X-Ray". These wavelengths also create burning, but usually we do not feel it until it is too late.

Both UVA and UVB affect the skin and age it. UVB burns the skin causing a toughening of the outer cells and a reaction in the melanin that we call tanning. The skin browns to create a sublevel barrier to protect the moisture balance and the health of the skin. UVA rays are the deeper penetrating rays that affect the deeper levels of the skin and attack the collagen as well as sneaking past the melanin protection barrier.

The UVB rays are our early warning system causing the skin to turn red and follows the same stages as a burn by fire or chemicals. This burning action tells us to get out of the sun or cover-up. The UVA, deep penetrating rays, do not have an early warning system beyond the UVB burning, so it is best to think of it as if it were nuclear radiation poisoning. The more you are exposed to the more you accumulate and the longer term it will affect you.

The National Cancer Institute says that 90% of all non-melanoma skin Cancers are associated with exposure to UV radiation from the sun. There is that 90% number again.

Even more interesting to me is the misconception we seem to have that people get all of our sun damage when we are young. Contrary to popular belief, 80 percent of a person's lifetime sun exposure is not acquired before age 18; only about 23 percent of lifetime exposure occurs by age 18.

Lifetime UV Exposure in the United States

Ages	Average Accumulated Exposure*
1-18	22.73 percent
19-40	46.53 percent
41-59	73.7 percent
60-78	100 percent

Many doctors tell me that when it comes to skin aging, that most of the damage happens in our early adult to mid-life years because of cumulative UVA damage and the chemo-aging process of just getting older. Ironically, they also tell me that the majority of skin cancer damage does come in the early teen years to young adulthood.

Jimmy Buffet wrote, "All of those sun baked tourists covered with oil" in his song "Margaritaville" about Key West in 1977. I spend a fair amount of time in Key West and some of those tourists are still there. Most are a nice shade of brown shoe leather.

Okay, it is time to put out those arms again! Now do see any difference between the tops and bottoms.

Bronze is Beautiful?

My wife Wendy is a classic old movie fan. We also have a lot of actors that are close friends. The commonality between these old movies and our actor friends? No Tans!

Yep! Tanning did not come into vogue until the 1930's, but hit full swing in the 60's and 70's with all those surfer movies.

Next time you are wandering through the movie channels and come across an old western or a desert epoch, notice that the people are all covered up. Big hats, long sleeves and often some sort of bandana or face covering. Common sense or beauty secret?

Universally when we talk with our actor friends, male or female, they have clear clean youthful skin. They quickly share that they make their living with their looks and that getting old looking is the curse of Hollywood.

I was sharing this little story with a customer while in a store in Santa Barbara and the woman quickly pointed out naming a couple of well-known actresses that had tans. I told her they were not tans! She looked puzzled and I said they are sprayed on! I really do not think she bought it because she took her dark brown-leathered skin body and left the store.

So where did all this start. Like the chemicals that started to invade our lives in the 1930's, so did tanning and sunglasses to create, "The Look."

Funny, sunglasses were supposedly invented on the movie set to protect actor's eyes from the bright lights. By 1929, a guy named Foster Grant widely popularized sunglasses as a fashion statement. Urban myth? I do not know, but it helps my story.

The other true story or myth is that tanning was started by Coco Chanel by accident. The way the story goes is that she was headed to

Cannes for the film festival on a nobleman's yacht and fell asleep in a deck chair. When she awoke, she was burned but quickly tanned. When she arrived at the film festival, she wore her sunglasses to not look like a raccoon and had this deep tan where other actors were light skinned. The look was born and so was the destruction of billions of skin cells.

Circa 1960's- 70's Tanning culture rides the wave

Picture a sun-drenched California beach with young muscle builders, beach babes and surfer dudes. Back then, the "Ho Daddy's" were actually the "wantabe" surfers that hung out on the beach, in hopes of cruising with the beach babes. The genuine surfers didn't care about all of the beach hubbub; after all they really just wanted to catch the perfect wave and hang ten.

No kidding—the tanning culture did not start in the U.S. until the 1960's. For the countless hours they spent outdoors in the sun, young people created the foundation for some extensive cumulative skin damage—radiation is real, it burns skin tissue. Skin that is tanned is the body's response mechanism to the repeated injury to their skin. Pictures of Hollywood stars on Malibu and Santa Monica beaches and poolside in Palm Springs and Las Vegas jump started the culture of tanning in this country. And unfortunately many of them today still continue to fuel the fire!

Interesting flashback...if you watch an old period movie on the Turner Classic Movie channel you are likely to see cowboys wearing long sleeved shirts, long pants and hats and gloves; while western frontier women appear with long skirts, long sleeved shirts, gloves, big brimmed hats and parasols. As if!

Not so long ago it really was all about taking cover from the sun and the elements. Well, I believe it is once again high time to take prudent cover and understand how to protect yourself and your loved ones every day of the year from damaging solar radiation.

Circa 2005 – The stakes are high

We are paying a huge price for continually damaging our skin

You are never too old or too young to suffer from the damaging effects of solar radiation. Scientific studies recently found that having several sunburns over the course of a lifetime can double or even triple melanoma risk, no matter when the sunburns occur. The fact is there are no safe ultraviolet (UV) rays or safe suntans.

More than half of all new cancers in the USA are skin cancers. The sun is responsible for more than 90 percent of all skin cancers. Precaution and early diagnosis could prevent 100,000 new cancer cases and 60,000 melanoma deaths in the U.S. each year!

The Mayo Clinic revealed in August 2005 that their studies have indicated that the incidence of two types of skin cancer has tripled in women under 40. Skin cancers are increasing rapidly in people over age 50 as well. Melanoma skin cancer is rising at an alarming rate.

Melanoma is dangerous because it can be a horrifyingly swift and silent killer if not detected at its earliest stages. There are many stories of heartbreak of losing loved ones so early in their lives to this type of cancer and leaving a legacy of the importance of being vigilant and paying attention to the skin's early warning signals. Early diagnosis is in fact the best chance for excellent cure rates.

The Secret to Youthful Healthy Skin! Cover up!

Much of this book is about chemicals in cosmetics and personal care products. This chapter is intended to save your youth and your life. Unlike the other chapters, this one is really not about chemicals in sunscreens. This chapter originally started with that as the topic, but this chapter bloomed to over twenty thousand words almost instantly. I decided that you probably already get the connection between chemicals and your skin health. So, I will leave it to the Environmental Working Group's Sun Screen Reports and maybe a book from Wendy to delve into what is safe and what is not. I do feel that I have to touch on the subject a bit and in a way that helps you.

Let's go back to UVA and UVB rays. It is very important to realize that the safest way to protect your youth and your skin health is to cover up with a big hat, UV sunglasses and UPF rated clothing wearing sun protection on exposed skin...usually the face, neck and hands.

Remember that those UVB rays burn and that UVA rays age. There are a few things that most people do not know.

1. The SPF rating on sunscreens does not rate UVA rays. The SPF or Sun Protection Factor started to emerge in 1962 and found national use in the 1970's.

2. To be safe, you need a sun protection product to be rated for both UVA and UVB.

3. UVA radiation penetrates car windows and building windows with most films designed to reduce UVB and infrared.

We know it is a fact that 90% of all visible skin aging is caused by sun damage. We have learned that 90%+ of skin Cancers are caused by sun damage. We also know that the only real way to protect our skin from UVA and UVB radiation is to cover up with clothing, hat, sunglasses and a broad-spectrum sunblock. What we do not know of is a chemical, natural or synthetic, that reverses sun damage. Also, more than 20 Americans die each day from skin Cancer.

I hope this is enough to convince you to research the effects and affects of UV radiation on your youth and your health.

Chapter Tools

1. 90% of all visible skin aging comes from sun exposure.

2. 90+ % of all skin cancer come from sun exposure.

3. There is no known way to reverse skin damage.

4. The best secret for youthful healthy skin is to cover up, with a UV rated hat, UV rated sunglasses, UV rated clothing and broad spectrum sun protection (sun block) on exposed skin.

5. Melanoma is deadly, so take it seriously.

Chapter 10: Who's Right?

"Most of us are graduates of MSU! We can go from nowhere to Making Shit Up in a nano-second. This is especially true in this internet age where opinion is in abundant quantity."

Bob Root

I really debated on this chapter being in the book because it just felt too negative to me. Then I thought that this book has morphed into a DIY How to book for people wanting to clean up their skin act. I realized that I spend as much time dispelling as I do educating. Almost daily, I get a note from our customer service people asking me to comment on some blog or chat forum about something someone said. These range from innocent mistakes people make to downright bold self-serving plagiarism. Worse are those that redo someone else's work with their own. Like the woman that writes for a national magazine that took the Marin County Cancer Projects 'Dirty Dozen' Chemicals and replaced many of them with her own and claimed that they were the original 'Dirty Dozen.'

There are those who also use sensationalism to raise money for their causes. I recall one that told their constituents that nano zinc oxide was unsafe sighting non-existent research and using weasel words to misdirect and change perception. With a glossary of over 400 studies to the contrary, I went on this group blog and threatened to build a mock cemetery in front of their building because of all the skin Cancer victims that die because of their efforts to raise money. They removed the article, but never retracted it.

Thinking of this, I realized that it is important for everyone to form their own opinion for what is good for them and not.

Because of my study of linguistics, I also realized that people are adept at using words like a magician uses sleight of hand. Ironically, sleight of hand, also known as prestidigitation or "quick fingers" seems an appropriate term since they use a keyboard instead of playing cards. I call these sleight of word master more appropriately FUD Masters. Where FUD stand for Fear, Uncertainty and Doubt! Clearly those that use fear, uncertainty and doubt to further their position of stature or position are suspect. Most of this takes on the form of innocent blogging and some, not so innocent. So, this chapter is not a rant, but a tool in creating your own life's database.

Further, this form of prestidigitation in blogging is so prolific that the US Federal Trade Commission enacted a law against bloggers and writers that gain monetarily from promoting or bashing products.

What really prompted this chapter?

I was contacted by one of our customers who is a regular user of our sunblock. She is a Melanoma survivor that told me that she stopped using our Solar Rx and all sunscreens because of something she read in a blog. The irony is that her fear had nothing to do with nano zinc or any other nano particles; it was because the writer was blasting companies that use vegetable emulsifying wax because they believe that all waxes are "all the same" contain undisclosed chemicals. Their claim: "We use a non-PEG emulsifier from the UK." Keys tested this non-PEG emulsifier and found the existence of other chemicals that precluded using them in our products. Irresponsible, Yes! Even more is that it is threatening this melanoma survivor's life based on FUD.

FUD or FACTS? STOP, Challenge and Choose.

Always follow your intuition when it comes to products, companies and people. Never let fear control you because as I define it, FEAR is really an acronym standing for **F**alse **E**xpectations **A**ppearing **R**eal

Negative marketing is just that..Negative! Look for the positive and I assure you that you will find it.

FUD vs. Facts, Blogging Not So Innocent

I spend 300 days a year on the road with our customers, retailers and at industry events. I receive numerous questions every day. The majority are inspiring and educational for me.

Almost daily though, I receive questions from people that relate to opinions expressed by some people or companies that are not based in fact and literally scare people. They conjure fear in people and I wonder what motivates these people to use negative marketing to further themselves or elevating themselves in other peoples' eyes.

We see both journalists and companies using fear tactics to try to sell themselves, their publications or their products. We call this the FUD factor. FUD stands for Fear, Uncertainty and Doubt and is the antitheses of facts. I see ads, blogs and opinions that border criminal because their comments will often scare people so badly that they stop using their prescription products that threatens their lives.

Ironically, negative and comparative marketing are illegal in Europe. Companies must sell their products based on the features, benefits and advantages and not a distinction based on what they do not have in their products. Companies and journalists that insight fears are held liable for their actions and comments. Yes, we are a free country and what we say as opinion is upheld by the constitution.

When I am on the road and answer peoples' questions, they usually ask me how they can weed out the facts from the FUD...negative marketing! I say it is easy.

In the Fight against FUD, here are a few suggestions:

When you hear someone or some company saying that their product does not contain an ingredient and that is why they do not use a particular ingredient! STOP, Challenge and Choose!

If you read an opinion expressed as if it were a fact without any stated! STOP Challenge and Choose!

If a product only claims what they do not have in them! STOP, Challenge and Choose!

If an article or product does not state a solution, but only negative perception! STOP, Challenge and Choose!

If your intuition tells you that what you are hearing is scary! STOP, Challenge and Choose!

What does STOP, Challenge and Choose mean?

STOP everything and do not fall victim to opinion without facts. Do not make anything up about what you are hearing, reading or feeling.

Challenge what people are saying or claiming and ask for studies, facts and detailed information so that you can make up your mind by balancing facts and opinion.

Choose your direction based on your intuition about people and their motives. Is it you they care about? Choose based on facts and not FUD.

There is a Sinister Side to the Internet

Sorry if this conflicts with some core beliefs, but because something is on the Internet does not mean it is correct!

The Federal Trade Commission (FTC), protects consumers from fraud or deceptive business practices, voted 4 to 0 to update its rules governing endorsements. The new guidelines require bloggers and celebrities to clearly disclose any "material connection" to and including payments for an endorsement or free product.

This is the first time since 1980 that the FTC has updated its rules on the use of endorsements and testimonials in advertising. In addition to covering bloggers, the new FTC rules state that celebrity endorsers can be held liable for false statements about a product, and all endorsements must include results consumers can "generally expect." Previously, an advertiser could cover their claims by the disclaimer "results not typical."

There is not a week that goes by that we receive a sort of "form letter" email from some blogger that threatens us that they will write a bad review of our products or company if we do not send free products. We usually respond by asking for an audit of their readership.

The new rules on bloggers are very far-reaching and appear to be attempting to create some guidelines of conduct. The past belief that inauthentic bloggers would suffer the fate of public opinion has not worked. We believe that this has not happened because most readers of blogs are voyeurs, which have allowed the "bad apples" to flourish.

The new rules went into effect December 1, 2009 and penalties include $11,000 in fines per violation. The FTC wasn't specific about how disclosures must be communicated but said its decisions would be made on a "case-by-case" basis.

Beginning December 2nd 2009 we began turning over those email extortions we receive to the FTC.

It covers everyone!

Specifically covered in the new rules is the use of social media, such as Twitter, by celebrities to endorse a product. That is now illegal and fineable unless the commercial relationship is disclosed. So, too, are celebrity mentions of products in other media, such as talk shows.

But the new rules on blogging will have the farthest-reaching influence. They are, in effect, the first rules imposed on a general public that no longer needs access to TV, print or radio to publish opinions or create a personal media channel.

The government agency has been reviewing its nearly 40-year-old rules on testimonials and endorsements for the better part of a year, and marketers have been anticipating a change.

Natural Products and Supplement Industry Big Culprits

There are numerous situations in the natural products and supplement industry that we believe helped spark this new ruling. The natural products industry has been growing in leaps and bounds compared to conventional products for more than five years. The Natural Product Association has seen spectacular growth even in recessive times. Many manufacturers seeking to maintain growth against new small upstart companies respond, not with new products or research, but with social marketing campaigns. There is an entire new breed of marketing agency that promotes "guerilla" campaigns in the social network sphere. Another nail in the coffin of so-called WOM/Guerilla/Buzz agencies!

We have actually experienced name brand companies support a position we take at a Safe Cosmetics Compact Signer meeting only to see them blogging against our position the next day. We now know that some companies have teams of hired bloggers to attack others as well as endorsing their new product launches.

Sinister sounding? Yes! Because it is!

Detecting Sinister Bloggers

Our customer service team has been squawking for us to write something about how some bloggers operate because they take the brunt of all of the emails when someone writes something that reflects on us or the industry. Daily, we get emails to our customer service that start with, "I heard that someone said that….and I am afraid that...and what do you think?" Thankfully, most of our customers know to write to us for information based on facts.

So, let's have some fun with this part. Rather than beating this into the ground, we decided to give the blogging styles of these bad guys' names and descriptions. These "types" are not just aimed at bloggers, but any advocacy group using each of these techniques to further their interests or to raise money to further their interests. I try to have some fun here with a very serious real situation that I believe harms the fabric of our society with misinformation.

In no particular order, these are the types of opinion-ators we see in the natural marketplace. Our purpose here is to give you a sense and the knowledge to detect. We hope it will help sharpen your antenna.

The "We" on themselves

I have heard that some bloggers act as if it is an entire team of people writing each of their opinions. As if a large group has more authority than a single writer. Most bloggers are lone individuals writing without collective input. What I look for are those credible sources that use their name or at least "I" in their posts. Someone that says, "I believe...or I think" rank high on our integrity meter.

The "No Comments"

This is one I love because I hate it so much. These blogs offer no place for you to comment on what they say. Yep, no button to click to add any opinion, bolster, refute or offer opinion on what they have said. These sites seem to live by the old adage of "from god's lips to their ears." I believe that if a blog does not offer a place to comment, you should not read what they are writing. Just "off" them. And certainly do not click the donation button. By the way, many blogs do have a time delay before your opinion shows because most have an approval cycle because there is another type of blogger that uses a quick opinion followed by a promotion of their own product or blog. They usually look something like this. "Great article and if you buy my weight reduction pill form my website www.urstuck.com ..."

The "They Said's"

Ioften get emails that substantiate a position with the term, "They Said." Who are they?

The "MyTwitFacers"

These are people that use all of their 140 characters to question, evoke, provoke or invoke some sort of reaction. Perhaps the new ruling will eliminate these types of bloggers because they will have to use most of their 140 characters to disclose that they are being paid to provoke, evoke and invoke.

The "FUD Factors"

I wrote previously all about FUD.

FUD stands for Fear Uncertainty and Doubt. When I used to read bloggers that create fear in people, I was just disgusted. It was when a young skin Cancer survivor told me that she was going to stop using sunscreen because she had read that she was afraid based on a blog article written by an influential NGO in Washington DC (not the EWG). My disgust turned to pure red-faced anger. Despite research study after research study, 400 in all, this scared Cancer survivor now was

142

endangering her life because of what some group had said. Sitting with her in a cafeteria at a natural food market near Dayton Ohio, I explained to her the risk and the science of why she needed clothing to cover as much of her skin as possible, while using sunblock on exposed skin. She and others like her were the inspiration and instigation of the number of sun protection articles I have written and as resolve for us to continue our skin Cancer advocacy.

If you are experience FUD, it feels first like Fear and if you search for any facts, the term FEAR is quickly realized that to stand for False Expectations Appearing Real.

In my humble opinion, like in many EU countries, FUD users should be fined and placed in jail. Furthering your own interests at the expense of others is wrong. Endangering their lives is criminal.

The "Fire Fire's"

A close relative to the FUD blogger is the Fire Fire Blogger. These people run from blog to blog yelling 'fire fire!' and then disappear. They will be the one where a blog is settling into a good stream of flow where people are openly contributing and then they will shoot some sort of blast that derails the dialog. Paid to do this. I think so!

The "Fake Facts"

This is the seasoned anti-blogger that quotes studies that don't exist or even worse alters a result of a study to substantiate an opinion. Hoping no one will research or even take the time to even check the study for accuracy, these blogger bend opinion with controversy based on lies.

The "Footnoters"

I find these blogs and articles humorous in a sort of strange engineering way.

As the story goes, I once had a professor that had us write a scientific paper where every noun had to have a footnote. Usually, he had us write papers of a certain word count, but in this case he did not specify how many words we were supposed to write. The topic we were supposed to write about was, "The origin of electricity." He told us that it was a project that his doctoral professor had assigned as preparation for his thesis. I and my fellow classmates struggled to write what we thought was supposed to be a 5,000 word essay with every word footnoted. It was painful and nearly impossible. I remember calculating that the essay was only worth 5% of my grade, so I bagged the project and turned in a blank page with the comment that my time was worth more than the grade. He laughed and accepted papers for everyone. Then he showed us his essay to his professor. To the question of "the origin of electricity?" It had a single word answer, God[1]... The footnote The Bible[1].

Sorry for the lengthy story, but I have seen one particular group write three different articles about three different subjects using the exact same footnotes in precisely the same order. A cut and paste? Clearly! The purpose? I suppose to make people think that they really studied for the article content.

The "Para-Plagiarists"

These amazing individuals have no original thoughts.

I have long been friends and advocates for the Marin County Cancer Project and their morphing into Search for the Cause. Early on I sought permission to republish their "Dirty Dozen" Chemical list and credit them in everything we write using the term. I believe that it is moral "trademarking" to honor those that created phrases or terms to help people in some way. Recently, I was directed to a blog by a customer asking why we used a "Dirty Dozen" chemical. When I went to the site, I was astounded that this blogger-writer had changed many of the chemicals to exclude the ones her product used and substituted others that competitive products were using on her list. The ingredient on her list that we used....Aloe! Yet our customer inquired and I was able to explain the lack of integrity. When I confronted the individual, her answer was, "I can say anything I want." No you can't when it is at the expense of others.

This sort of marketing was also recently tested by a lawsuit launched by Dr Bronner's against a number of companies over the "Organic Seal" they had on their products. These companies chose to bend the term "organic" in some way or another to cause Dr Bronner's to take legal action based on damaging their business. The detail of the case is on their website, but the point herein is that people that blog for their own gain at the expense of others is not against the new FTC ruling, but it is against the law.

The "Dumb Chills"

Dumb chills are what you get when someone does something so stupid that it gives you chills!

We read them all the time in blogs where someone gets something so wrong that they appear so stupid that you never click on their site ever again. Unfortunately, they keep writing and influencing first time…hopefully only time visitors.

As an example, we were going to a pet trade show in Las Vegas. Before the show exhibitors prepare a short, 150 word, description of what people can see at their booth for publication in the show program. In our case, we were in a new section of the show called Natures Pathway indicating the first section of the show dedicated to natural products. So, in our description we wrote that our pet products contained no Sodium Laureth Sulfate (SLS) and was based on a terrible experience we had with our pup and a brand of shampoo that nearly killed him because it had so much SLS.

So, we show up at the show and on opening day we walk by this booth with a giant sign that says No Sodium Chloride (table salt). I have to admit that I did not understand what that meant or why they would put up such a sign. One of our dealers went and asked them what that meant and the company owner said, "we are natural too just like those Keys people, we don't use salt either"…Sodium Laureth Sulfate …not sodium chloride… Dumb Chills!

Even though it is a tradeshow story, I commonly see people and companies in their blogs saying really dumb things. Not against the new FTC ruling or the law in general. Just dumb and scary that people listen the way they do.

Not convinced? I have been CNN free for over ten years. When I have been exposed to CNN in an airport or outside a convention, I am astounded at what they are saying labeled as fact and is clearly opinion. Many of the blogs I read present opinion in such an arrogant way that expect me to believe them in such a way that it gives me dumb chills. In most cases, these are blogs that do not offer a comment box.

The "Seals of Approval"

Did you know that the Skin Cancer Foundation, of which we are members, requires an upfront investment of tens of thousands of dollars to be considered for a seal of approval. This to me seems like a paid product endorsement. Many other organizations also require deep cash investments, sometimes annually, to gain their endorsement. As a consumer, what you see is a seal on your sunscreen that comes from the Skin Cancer Foundation or the American Dermatological Society etc., thinking that it is some sort of quality endorsement. Not realizing that it is purchased.

Many blogs tout certifications, memberships and endorsement as justification of their opinion. Indeed we even do this to some extent in our compliance with Safe Cosmetics and the EWG. It is when you use these certifications to justify what you do it is stepping over the boundaries of good practices.

The "Negatives"

Unfortunately some companies use negative blogging, marketing and advertising to drag down others and competitors rather than improving their own products or marketing the features, benefits and advantages of what they offer. Blogging, talking and writing why others are bad and comparing negative aspects is categorically illegal in the EU, but not in the US. Dragging down a company, product or individual does not elevate that individual in my eyes. There is a phrase in Japanese that translates to "When the nail sticks up we must pound it down." Basically translated to me that to keep society on an even foundation, individuals that stick out should be shown their place by society. Negative marketing only serves to elevate or normalize everyone by trying to pound down the products that jump to a lead through innovation. Believe this or not, there are entire advertising agencies that tout, promote and market themselves to blast companies and their products in a negative way. Illegal? No! Immoral?

Conclusion

I spend about half of my week on the internet writing, reading and offering my opinion on blogs, forums and chat areas. Much is within the technical community, but a lot on consumer and industry forums. First, I use my real name! I learn a great deal and offer opinion. Over the last five years, I have seen the characters I describe above grow to an alarming level. Often undetected, I commonly refer to them collectively as "Underground Bunnies". Often cute, fuzzy looking bloggers with ill intent, they use words that manipulate with questionable intent. They operate underground for the sole purpose of self.

Granted that what I am talking about here might appear semi-remote or disconnected from the FTC ruling. I think not! If you imagine that some sources estimate that 30% of bloggers talking about products are paid to do so, then what techniques do they use to get your attention and swing your opinion? I suggest the ones above are most common and the techniques are diverse and dynamic as there are paid bloggers.

I see this ruling as powerful and debilitating as was the crack-down on those guys that call you at dinner time. These bloggers are the same and with even more sinister intent.

I am excited about the new FTC ruling because it will level the ground and hopefully reverse this bad trend.

Am I over reacting to a small thing? I don't think so. Keep in mind that the government...the FTC did step in and did something about it. How bad is it? The government acted, so it must really be bad. Worse than I even know or describe.

And it all happened without Michael Moore making a movie about it.

Chapter 11: Scary Chemical That Begin with the Dirty Dozen

Our skin health is based on balance, nutrition and the products we use. Upset that balance in any way and the skin is a quick victim.

Lets me explain what I am talking about with another story.

A few years ago, I was helping a friend of mine work on a documentary about a new surgical procedure and instrument that he had invented. Technologically it was very cool for its time and I had some time to help him document the features and functions of the instrument as well as his special procedure.

I spent a lot of hours in the operating room with him holding a video camera attached to the device as he performed surgeries. In the process, I met a large number of surgeons who visited to learn the procedure first hand. Hand being the key word!

What I noticed was that when shaking their hand, every surgeon that I met had rough crusty cracked hands. This was a long time before starting Keys, but I recall asking them why. All complained that it was the antibacterial soap that they had to use. I was curious and snagged one of these disposable little sterile packed brush and sponge combos that had the soap built in. The docs would pop open the paper pouch and scrub from their fingertips to their elbow. Then a sterile drape before donning surgical gloves made mostly from latex.

The lead chemical in this little cleaning apparatus was hexachlorophene . Later, science discovered that Hexachlorophene could be lethal from absorption through the skin. Oh well, you get the point I hope.

Their hands were a wreck so that they could protect their patients from bacteria and germs.

When we started Keys, it was after developing the products for Wendy's sensitive skin. We never used any of the Dirty Dozen chemicals because each seemed to have a personal reaction for Wendy. In her case and the development of our products, simple whole natural ingredients that functioned the way she needed were our only choice.

As a side note, it is important for you to remember that most of the product brands you see on a store shelf come from a few companies that provide base products as contract manufacturers. The individual brands usually alter their perception to users via a fragrance or packaging with a few differentiated ingredients thrown in here and there. This is the reason we built our own factory to make the product we wanted and needed. Contract manufacturers were not interested in my recipes!

If we had gone through a contract manufacturer, like an estimated 85% of the brands on store shelves, we would have had all the same ingredients as others struggling to differentiate on store shelves.

All this is important to keep into perspective when you are buying products.

For grins, just stand one day in your local natural products store in the personal care area and notice how many people unscrew the cap of a product and smell it. I will save you the trouble; it is half of the people.

The reason I bring this up is that we are conditioned this way by the manufacturers offering the exact same shampoo in 15 different fragrances.

Worse, when we think we do not want any fragrance, we reach for the unscented label. Sorry, but the industry has an entire field of chemistry to develop masking fragrance to make that product odorless.

This leads me to a quick description of the Dirty Dozen chemicals. I present this list here as not the end, but the beginning of your chemical sleuthing. As I mentioned before, there is already the 'Dirty Thirty' list and I saw another author refer to the 'Dirty 100'.

The reason I cover this here is simply to give you an idea where the chemicals are used, what they do and the concern that they cause. Think of this as a sort of format for your database.

The Dirty Dozen chemical list was first developed by the Marin County Cancer Project. Marin County California has experienced some of the highest cancer rates in America. They published this list of chemicals to educate people about the potential for cumulative toxic exposure to multiple chemicals in everyday products. They call them the "Dirty Dozen." You can read more at http://www.SearchfortheCause.org

The "Dirty Dozen" Chemicals in Everyday Products

At Keys, we believe that over 50% of all skin disorders for people and pets are misdiagnosed and are actually caused by chemicals in everyday products. In fact, over 95+% of all skin and pet care shampoos, bath gels, conditioners, laundry detergents and cosmetics contain one or more of these chemicals.

Notice the chemical name, its function, who uses it and the health concern. Then to start, take this list and match it against the products you have in your medicine cabinet, shower, under your sink or in the laundry. It may startle you how many products you use every day. It will even startle you more of how many contain these chemicals.

So here are the Dirty Dozen!

Sodium Laureth/Sodium Lauryl Sulfate

Function: Penetration enhancer

Present in: Shampoo/conditioner, bar soap, body wash, face cleanser, liquid hand soap, acne treatment, hair dye, mascara, shaving products, moisturizer, bar soap, toothpaste, sunscreen, makeup remover, perfume, cologne

Health Concern: Alters skin structure, allowing other chemicals to penetrate deep into the skin, increasing the amounts of other chemicals that reach the bloodstream.

Parabens (methyl, ethyl, propyl and butyl parabens)

Function: Parabens are a group of chemicals widely used as preservatives in cosmetics to inhibit bacteria, yeast and mold growth and are antibacterial agents in antibacterial toothpaste

Present in: Shampoos, conditioners, hair styling gels, nail creams, foundations, facial masks, skin creams, and deodorants, baby lotions, and other personal care products for children

Health Concern: May alter hormone levels, possibly increasing risks for certain types of Cancer, impaired fertility, or alteration of the development of a fetus or young child. May cause skin irritation, rash or dermatitis. or allergic skin reactions.

Propylene Glycol

Function: Penetration enhancer; keeps products from melting in high heat or freezing when it is cold

Present in: Shampoo/conditioner, bar soap, body wash, face cleanser, liquid hand soap, acne treatment, hair dye, shaving products, moisturizer, makeup remover, toothpaste, sunscreen, perfume, cologne, deodorant, toner/astringent, foundation, bronzer powder, nail polish, lip products, eye shadow/pencil, mascara

Health Concern: Alters skin structure, allowing other chemicals to penetrate deep into the skin, increasing the amounts of other chemicals that reach the bloodstream; skin irritant, causes allergic reactions.

Phthalates

Function: A family of industrial chemicals that are used as solvents in cosmetics

Present in: Nail polish, deodorant, fragrance, hair spray, hair gel/mousse, lotions

Health Concern: Phthalates can damage the liver, kidneys, lungs and in particular the developing male reproductive tract: Permanent birth defects in the male reproductive system.

Petrolatum

Function: Lubricant to make lipsticks shine and creams smoother; helps to soften skin in the same way as other products but much cheaper

Present in: Cold creams, lotions, wax depilatories, eyebrow pencils, eye shadows, liquid powders, lipsticks, protective creams, baby creams

Health Concern: May be contaminated with impurities, linked to Cancer or other significant health problems; causes allergic reactions.

Cocamide DEA/Lauramide DEA

Function: Used as foaming agents in shampoos and bath products, and as emulsifying agents in cosmetics; foaming and cleansing agent for "mouth feel"

Present in: Shampoo, Body Wash/Cleansers, Bath Oils, Facial Cleanser, Liquid Hand Soap, Bar Soap, Acne Treatment, Baby Wash, Shaving Products, Body Scrubs, Foot Odor/Cream Treatment, Deodorant, Moisturizer, Hair Dye/Spray

Health Concern: May be contaminated with impurities linked to Cancer or other significant health problems. May form carcinogenic compounds called nitrosamines on the skin or in the body after absorption. Insufficient toxicity data to determine safety in products that will be inhaled, where chemicals become airborne and can be inhaled.

Diazolidinyl Urea

Function: Formaldehyde-releasing, anti-microbial preservative

Present in: Moisturizer, Styling Products, Shampoo/conditioner, Hair Spray/Dyes, Anti-Aging Treatment, Facial Cleanser, Sunscreen, Facial Moisturizer, Foundation, Eye Makeup, Acne Treatment, Mascara, Body Wash/Cleansers, Deodorant, Concealer, Exfoliator, Powder, Body Scrubs, Bath Oils/Salts, Eye Contact Care, Lip Makeup, Shaving Products, After Sun Product, Douche/Personal Cleanser, Makeup Remover Depilatory Cream/Hair Remover, Liquid Hand Soap, Nail Treatments, Pain Relief Rub/Ointment, Fragrance

Health Concern: May be contaminated with impurities linked to Cancer or other significant health problems.

Butyl Acetate

Function: Solvent in polishes and treatments, prevents chipping

Present in: Nail polish and nail treatments like strengtheners, hardeners, top/base coats

Health Concerns: Repeated exposure causes skin dryness and cracking; vapors may induce drowsiness or dizziness.

Butylated Hydroxytoluene

Function: Anti-oxidant; slows down the rate at which product ingredients change in color

Present in: Lip Makeup, Moisturizer, Eye Makeup, Anti-Aging Treatment, Foundation, Fragrance, Bar Soap, Shaving Products, Antiperspirant/Deodorant, Concealer, Sunscreen, Facial Cleanser, Body Wash, Blush, Shampoo, Conditioner, Acne Treatment, Body Lotion/Oil, Powder, Makeup Remover, Depilatory Cream, Toothpaste, Styling Product, Exfoliator, Nail Treatments

Health Concern: Eye and skin irritant.

Ethyl Acetate

Function: Solvent

Present in: Nail polish products, mascara, tooth whitening, perfume

Health Concern: Eye and skin irritant.

Toluene

Function: Solvent to improve adhesion and gloss

Present in: Mainly nail polish and hair dye

Health Concern: Potentially Cancer causing, pregnancy concern, liver damage, irritating to the skin and respiratory tract; harmful by inhalation.

Triethanolamine

Function: A coating ingredient for fresh fruits and widely used as a dispersing ingredient in hand and body lotions, shaving cream, soaps; shampoos and bath powders.

Present in: Hand and body lotions, shaving creams, soaps, shampoos and bath powders

Health Concern: May form carcinogenic compounds called nitrosamines on the skin or in the body after absorption (compounds formed when chemicals containing nitrites react with amine, natural chemicals found in food and the body) -- among the most potent Cancer-causing agents found. Thought to possibly cause Cancer in humans, based on limited data.

Breaking It Down

Much of what stalled this book was the ever changing dynamics of the industry. Whether it is the definition of natural or organic, the dynamics of change seemed insurmountable until I backed away from the idea of listing all the chemicals out there and expressing a concern for each. What I decided to do is to create this book to give you some general guidelines to follow that would not date the book. Also, everywhere I turn, there are new chemicals being listed of concern as well as new research.

The Dirty Dozen are now the Dirty 30 and more than likely the Dirty 300 by the time this book sees the shelves. What I will try to explain herein are some things to consider. I will focus on some brief generalities and then pick a couple of chemicals that are of personal concern.

Many green chemists, activists and naturopaths express concern over the safety of many chemicals. Pick any one, Google it and you will be bombarded with opinion. My reasons for not using some chemicals are more functional and pragmatic.

SLS *Sodium Laureth/Lauryl Sulfate*

For example, Sodium Laureth Sulfate (SLS) and its 280 synonyms are said to be a concern from a public safety perspective. Yes, I know that it was originally designed as an engine degreasing concoction that works very well to suds in all types of hard or soft water. It is especially effective in washing hair to get all the grease out. When you look at the toxicity data on the National Institutes of Health (NIH) Toxnet database, it shows concerns in concentration and is considered harmful to humans in high concentrations.

For example, many laundry detergents use SLS to clean fabrics in our washing machines. The percentage is not listed on the labels, but we have measured the Top 10 brands and have found SLS levels in excess of 35%. Testing some HE versions are even higher. According to the documents at NIH these level are excessive, but manufacturers claim that they are being rinsed away in the rinse cycle. You may intuitively have a sense of this high SLS concentration. Many people I have met explain that they are running a double rinse of all of all of their laundry!

SLS is in most all personal care and home products that are designed to clean. Predominately used in shampoo and facial cleansers, it is also in toothpaste and some food. That dishwashing soap also has high levels of SLS to dissolve grease. Again, we do not necessarily know the levels of SLS as consumers because there is no requirement to list the ingredient or their amount on packaging.

Is it bad or is it good? Some say SLS is not harmful in small doses. Some say that it is not harmful at all. My reasons for not using SLS is that in testing and research we found that SLS makes the skin more permeable. Good thing or bad thing? I found that some manufacturers use SLS in those stop smoking and diet patches you wear on your arm. I was told it helps the medicine get into the skin more readily. Makes sense, I guess. I suspect that it could make the skin more susceptible to bacteria and other chemicals and that this could be a concern.

For me, the reason I do not use SLS is that in my tests on me and a few other engineers, we saw inflammation on the skin. We speculate that this sort of inflammation can be causing all sorts of diagnosed skin disorders. Docs have a code word for this which we found out is called Contact Dermatitis. I believe that it also has something to do with the epidemic of balding in men as well as some other skin disorders that carry the same diagnosis. We do know that inflammation is a big issue when it comes to bacteria, fungus and germs affecting the skin. Still, some claim that it is not harmful, but to my knowledge, there are no clinical trials testing SLS.

All of these chemicals have concern based on research and linked occurrences to disease and disorders. So profound it enabled Search for the Cause to be permitted to publicly link them to increased Cancer rates in their county.

All said, what scare the hell out of me are two very specific widely used chemicals in personal care and cosmetics. These are parabens and Triclosan. To me, they are simply Biocides that are indiscriminate killers creating super bugs.

Early in the book, I told you about how the skin works. Overly simplifying a particular facet of the skin, the bacteria that exist on it keep our skin in balance. Washing our skin and particularly the face removes the remnants of the bacteria, dirt, pollutants and dead skin. No matter how hard we try to remove the bacteria, it is nearly impossible unless we use germicides or bactericides like parabens and Triclosan.

Here is my simple concern. If I can put a paraben in a product to kill off bacteria and germs in the container, what does it do to the good bacteria on my skin? If I wash my hands with a hand sanitizer that contains the broad-spectrum bactericide, Triclosan, what does it do to my good bacteria?

Search as I might, I have not found any evidence that parabens and Triclosan are discrete killers. Meaning that they waste the bad guys and protect the good. Everything that I have read supports the contrary.

I have talked to dermatologists, doctors and scientists asking their concerns about what is going on in personal care and cosmetics that concern them. Over 90% express concern over parabens and Triclosan because of the long-term health effects. Not from the chemicals, but from the effect it has on killing the probiotics of our skin. All express an even greater concern about these chemicals being used in our food, toothpaste and mouthwashes.

You can choose to read this chapter or not. It is somewhat geeky, but necessary to explain my perceptions.

What I believe is that the only chemicals used in personal care known that kills the good bacteria on our skin are parabens and Triclosan. Remove the good bacteria and our balance is disrupted. Disrupt the balance and those bacteria that come at us first are the worst kind and literally attack unprotected skin.

I personally believe that these two chemical types are responsible for many of the skin disorders that doctors see.

It took western medicine a long time to buy into the fact that we need probiotics to help our gut perform. I believe it is also now time that we start to explore probiotics for our skin.

Finally, I do believe that the people that have link MRSA (Methicillin-Resistant Staphylococcus Aureus) outbreaks to parabens and Triclosan are probably correct. Only time and research will prove them right or wrong. Indications are they are correct and it is probably time to eliminate parabens and Triclosan from your life.

So read on if you want!

Triclosan: The Biocide that Creates Super Bugs?

FACT vs FUD is a chapter in this book as well as an article on our blog. In this overly inflammatory news based society of ours, my resistance is to publish anything that is not based in research that is a bit beyond a theory.

Some History:

One of the inspirations for this book and this article was an experience I had while in a store outside of Dayton Ohio. I was not too far from the headquarters of Proctor & Gamble (Cincinnati) delivering a speech about the Dirty Dozen at an annual event the store promotes. Probably 200 in attendance, I went through the Dirty Dozen chemicals created by the Marin County Cancer Project. At the end, I provided some chemicals of concern, so I went back through my "most feared" list. In the book, I describe that some of the Dirty Dozen are much more damaging than others are, but tend to be used in only discrete segments and in only some products. Some ingredients like parabens are much more widely used often in multiple doses during the manufacturing process elevating their concentrations in products to well beyond the called for percentages by the chemical maker. During my speech, I invited questions as we went along and there were plenty.

At the end, I voiced my concern that Triclosan was perhaps my greatest fear because it is so powerful a biocide. I had explained earlier that Triclosan is the main ingredient in hand sanitizers and antibacterial soaps. A biocide, by design, kills gram positive and gram negative bacteria as well as most all bacteria. My concern all along has been two very important concerns:

1. If it indiscriminately kills all bacteria, then what does it do to the flora-probiotic on our skin?

2. Will the destruction of all bacteria on the skin create super-bugs that morph and become resistant to both the biocide and antibiotics?

As I always do when speaking to a group, I try to connect with the eyes of people in my audience. It is my way of trying to figure out if I am connecting with them. In my corporate life, I received training on how to read an audience as well. As I call it, 'Squirming Around' is a big flag that I have touched a nerve. As a CEO of a publicly traded company, you had better believe that I experienced this at every shareholder meeting. So, this day, I was thrust back to my corporate life by a gentleman that had asked no questions, been very polite and had friendly eyes. When I lumped Triclosan in with parabens as my major concern, his hand shot skyward as to immediately interrupt me. I obliged by stopping to acknowledge his question.

He asked, "Why would you add the main ingredient in hand sanitizers with that of preservatives used in almost every product made from personal care, to toothpaste, to food?"

First things first, I knew immediately that this person was from the industry because the question was one I would have expected in a meeting inside a research and development process. Not being ever deterred by confrontation, I answered both technically and emotionally. Here is my initial response.

"I am more concerned with Triclosan than a Methyl Paraben for four primary reasons:

1. Triclosan has been used in hospital and scientific environments for many years because it is the most effect biocide.

2. The concentration of Triclosan in a function specific product like antibacterial soaps is much higher and therefore of greater concern to me because it does a much more wide reaching job of killing all bacteria on the skin including the good bugs!

3. The destruction from Triclosan is so powerful and long lived compare to parabens that I have more than a subtle concern that what bacteria arrive back on the scene will be the worst kind like staph, e. Coli etc.

4. I also worry that these strains of bacteria will grow back with a vengeance and become resistant to both Triclosan and known antibiotics."

The man stood straight up as if to confront me. I could also tell that I had just scared the hell out of the rest of the audience. Before I could temper my comments with the fact that this was my personal concern and that I had not gathered all the facts, he spoke.

He said, "I am a scientist that works down the road. First, I am a parent and father. I do not care that we have the best health insurance; I worry about what we expose our kids to. We have had an outbreak of Staph in the middle schools in this area and what you are saying is that because we require our kids to wash with antibacterial soap containing Triclosan that we are exposing them to the potential of transmitted staph infections like the ones we are experiencing now?"

My only answer had to be from the heart and not my corporate training to dodge the question. I said, Yes!"

He shook his head and sat down. Honestly, you could have heard a mouse burp in that room! I tried to interject some humor and my time was up. The people filed out of the room as the other speaker got set up. The man approached as did the sponsors from the store.

The sponsor thanked me for the informative talk and quickly said, can you send me something about this. She offered that she was a Cancer survivor and had a more than passing concern.

The man also echoed by adding that he was privileged to be able to read many documents about uses of chemicals. He said that what he always noticed is that most have warnings of irritation when used in high percentages and that antibacterial soap using Triclosan actually exceeded the minimum percentages. I asked if he could provide me with percentage data and he said; "No! I am not allowed to do that!" I got the message. I walked back to my team that was exhibiting at the health fare and told them of the experience. I shared, that I only wish I had a study to hand to everyone that at least echoed my fears.

Over the last two years, I have shared the story with colleagues. This morning in July of 2010, I received an email with a copy of the Opinion from the EU Scientific Directorate! Being a geek, I read all 56 pages and decided to sit down to finish this chapter of the book.

Remember this is an opinion and I would encourage you to read the entire document. There must be additional testing. We do know that bacteria exposed to destructive agents does morph into "super bugs" in many cases. This opinion echoes much of that concern. In one sense, I am pleased that this concern of mine and others has now taken another step up in the process of science.

My opinion! For what it is worth, science generally follows an orderly path. The Mandelbrot theory says that, if that what we see occurs in a large scale, it will occur in a small scale. If we can kill bacteria...good and bad... with a large dose of a chemical, then small doses delivered more frequently and repeatedly will have the same effect. The other scientific principle that comes to mind here is Occam's Razor which is the principle that "entities must not be multiplied beyond necessity" or that the simplest explanation is usually the correct one. To me it makes sense from a logical perspective that using a chemical like Triclosan everyday in large does will have a long term adverse effect on the flora of the skin. Only the test of time and scientific studies will bring the concern to even higher levels.

What I can share is that I personally avoid anything on or in my body designed to kill something like germs, bacteria and microbes. Like all of us, I have had to take antibiotics and we know from the warnings that sustained use can make them ineffective. Following Occam's Razor, I also believe that is true of these chemicals under various names that are designed to make my life more pure...Purity at the sake of what?

So, my mother may not have been right that eating dirt was all that bad for me ☺

Triclosan: The Biocide that keeps on giving!

Most of the free world including the US requires that Triclosan be listed somewhere on the label if it is used in a product. But how about if it is used in product packaging or molded into materials. Unregulated therefore no requirement for listing. Herein is the fallacy of confusing consequence with sequence.

Have you ever wondered why cheese seems to last longer than it used to? Have you wondered how companies can claim that if you buy their storage products that food will last longer? Have you wondered how a manufacturer could claim that their running socks are antibacterial?

We know that Triclosan is used in sanitizers and toothpaste as well as antibacterial soaps. Did you ever wonder what chemical they use in making utensils, cooking equipment, cutting boards and even sport clothing to make them antibacterial. You guessed it, Triclosan. The white powdery substance can be molded into products to make virtually antibacterial. Many food packages are molded with Triclosan to make them antibacterial to preserve the food longer.

If there was any reason to buy organic and local at the farmers market, this is a darned good one for me.

Like phthalates, Triclosan is not just in personal care. They found phthalates in children's toys and car dashboards.

Triclosan is in much more than antibacterial soap. Here is a partial list of products that use Triclosan:

- Sanitizers
- Antibacterial soap (really a detergent)
- Deodorant
- Toothpaste
- Shaving Cream
- Mouthwash
- Skin Care
- Makeup
- Acne Products
- Antimicrobial Creams
- Cleaning Supplies
- Kitchen Utensils
- Food Storage
- Plastic Wrap
- Trash Bags
- Toys
- Bedding (People and Pets)
- Socks
- Sports Clothing
- Child Car Seats

Someone asked me if I could link a direct connection to MRSA (Methicillin Resistent Staphylococcus Aureus) and Triclosan. I said, "Honestly, I do not know!" Do I believe that it is connected? Yes! So you can imagine my surprise when I read an article in a medical journal prescribe sits baths for MRSA suffers in a solution of 2% Tricolsan!

Triclosan is used in many common household products that you would not expect.

OK, I am starting to sound like a radical working at an NGO! Environmental issues are big as well.

Parabens...Good Guys or Bad Guys?

As a part of my ongoing series of looking at the Dirty Dozen Chemicals shown to provide elevated Cancer rates in people and animals, in this article, I outline why we do not use parabens leaving the judgmental diagnosis to the NGO's attacking them. The Dirty Dozen Chemicals are a list of 12 developed originally by the Marin County Cancer Project that at the time, had the highest Cancer Rates in the US. Followed by Search For The Cause and Teens Turning Green the list is now designated the Dirty Thirty.

So, are parabens good guys or bad guys? Both it seems and there is a reason why we do not use them as well.

Below is a scavenged description of parabens from Wikipedia. On the surface and from a chemical perspective they do their job. Many chemists and companies support their use based on a belief of safety. I believe that they are looking at the wrong reasons for safety.

Our society seems to primarily look at safety as, "will what we put on our skin hurt us directly?" I believe that we should be looking at whether it hurts us based on contact and will it cause something else to hurt us because of it.

So first, let's try to understand what parabens are and why some manufacturers use them. Here is that Wikipedia description:

Parabens are a class of chemicals widely used as preservatives in the cosmetic and pharmaceutical industries. Parabens are effective preservatives in many types of formulas. These compounds, and their salts, are used primarily for their bactericidal and fungicidal properties. They can be found in shampoos, commercial moisturizers, shaving gels, personal lubricants, topical/parenteral pharmaceuticals, spray tanning solution and toothpaste. They are also used as food additives.

Their efficacy as preservatives, in combination with their low cost, their long history of safe use and the inefficacy of natural alternatives like grapefruit seed extract (GSE), probably explains why parabens are so commonplace. They are becoming increasingly controversial, however, and some organizations which adhere to the precautionary principle object to their everyday use.

Chemistry

Parabens are esters of *para*-hydroxy*benz*oic acid, from which the name is derived. Common parabens include methylparaben , ethylparaben, propylparaben and butylparaben. Less common parabens include isobutylparaben, isopropylparaben, benzylparaben and their sodium salts.

Occurrence

Some parabens are found naturally in plant sources. For example, methylparaben is found in blueberries, where it acts as an antimicrobial agent. However, when parabens are eaten, they are metabolized and lose the ester group, making them less strongly estrogen-mimicking.

(Bob Comment) Part of the rub here is a number of studies that link parabens to breast Cancer because of these properties, but let's not get too off track!

Synthesis

All commercially used parabens are synthetically produced, although some are identical to those found in nature. They are produced by the esterification of *para*-hydroxybenzoic acid with the appropriate alcohol. *para*-Hydroxybenzoic acid is in turn produced industrially from a modification of the Kolbe-Schmitt reaction, using potassium phenoxide and carbon dioxide.

Now that you are an expert on parabens, I think it is fair to talk about the pros and cons of them.

Remember that I believe that it is an indirect result of the parabens that is as important to look at as well as the direct result of their actions.

The pros of parabens or grapefruit seed extract are that they kill bacteria and fungus inside products. It is very difficult to sterilize containers and apparatus without using chemicals. The technique we use is super-heated steam on our equipment, but those parabens do a good job of killing microbes, gram positive and gram-negative rods.

The con is that they do a good job of killing bacteria on our skin as well.

You might say that is good, but much research shows that what we want to do is inhibit bacteria growth on our skin while permitting flora bacteria to exist as it does in nature. To me, it is sort of like drinking parabens in hope they will kill diseased bacteria in our gut in hopes that they will leave all that good bacteria we want alone. If science could figure that out, it would be major... just has not happened yet.

Frankly, when I developed our first products, I did not know what parabens were. So it was simple...ignorance was bliss. I did know that I needed a preservative and my aboriginal friends suggested rosemary. Turns out it is also a natural high-grade antioxidant, but for me, it minimized bacteria growth in our natural products.

When a contract manufacturer approached me to make our products, I politely listened as the salesperson told me why I had to use parabens. My silence forced him to exasperation and he blurted out, "What would you do if the FDA said you have to use parabens?" My answer? I would mark the products refrigerate after opening! He was not amused and yet that is exactly what I would do.

It turns out that we have traced part of Wendy's reaction to prescription products after her Melanoma to a paraben reaction. Admittedly rare, I personally believe that it is more common than we think.

I will let our friends at the Breast Cancer Fund fight the paraben battle on their own front. I would encourage you to research that more for yourself.

Why We Do Not Use Parabens

Simply, I have done enough research and read enough that parabens in our personal care, household products and mouth care kill all forms of bacteria on our skin and in our gut. Like studies have shown with Triclosan and germicides used in household products, my own studies have shown these same agents kill the natural flora on the skin and in the gut. What I believe happens next is that the really bad bacteria including gram positive rods like e. Coli and Staph (MRSA) have an opportunity to come back with a vengeance and attack our systems freely.

For example, it is common in our microbiology lab to take an agar Petri dish and smear a natural ingredient on it to see if colony, gram positive or gram negative rods (bacteria) show up in an accelerated 72 hour test. What is not common, but we have done it, are to take a sample of "bugs" and kill them and then watch what grows back first in an open-air environment. More than not, we see some harmless colony bacteria show up first, but then some really nasty bacteria take over and on most occasions we see fungus appear to feed on the bacteria. Can't prove it, but I have to wonder if all this MRSA staph that has shown up in our middle schools is not a direct link to the Triclosan in antibacterial soaps and the parabens in all of our products.

Okay, now that I have you flipped out a bit, I did a test of ten products at one of my labs and measured the cumulative amount of parabens in them. What I mean is that I know that the providers of parabens suggest a range or percentage to use. Let's say it is 0.5% of the total solution. When I tested the products all showed excessive amounts of parabens well beyond the recommended dose. Knowing that chemists strive for economy, I began to wonder why the levels were so high...high enough to kill anything. I could not figure out why until I was giving a speech on the Dirty Dozen near Dayton Ohio and one chemist from P&G asked how many ingredients were typically in natural products. I answered, "probably 10 to 15." He laughed and said our average is 45. It suddenly dawned on me how the paraben levels could be so high in the products I tested. The answer, the ingredient/chemical suppliers were also using parabens to preserve their raw material. Think it through! The manufacturer puts 0.5% into the product and each of the suppliers of those 40+ chemicals put 0.5% into the raw materials. Simply, we are being overdosed with parabens and every product we use adds to the equation. Ten products times the 1.6% average we tested is a daily dose of 16% on our skin. I think the most recent statistics I heard from the EWG is that the average woman uses 12 products a day containing parabens and men average 6 products. That means that if I am correct with my average that women are getting ~19.2% paraben contact. We have always joked that "chemists add and engineers subtract, but maybe it is not a joke.

Our Simple View

The reason we do not use parabens is that we believe that what comes out of the bottle designed to kill bacteria in the packaging also kills the flora on our skin and our gut facilitating bad super-bug bacteria to grow in its place that also facilitates fungal growth and imbalance.

Right now, this is a tested theory long from scientific fact. What if I am right!

See, I told my mother eating dirt was good!

BTW, The Mayo Clinic states, *"Most MRSA infections occur in hospitals or other health care settings, such as nursing homes and dialysis centers. It's known as **health care-associated MRSA, or HA-MRSA.** Older adults and people with weakened immune systems are at most risk of HA-MRSA. More recently, another type of MRSA has occurred among otherwise healthy people in the wider community. This form, **community-associated MRSA, or CA-MRSA,** is responsible for serious skin and soft tissue infections and for a serious form of pneumonia."*

I personally believe that people are walking in with the MRSA and when surgery is performed that is when it invades. Maybe hospitals should pretest for MRSA and an incoming inspection....Do you think?

Chapter Tools

1. Parabens and Triclosan are bactericides and germicides. That means they kill bacteria and germs.

2. Parabens and Triclosan indiscriminately kill the good probiotic bacteria on the skin. My belief is that this permits bad bacteria attacking the undefended skin.

3. Washing the skin does not remove our probiotic good bacteria from the skin.

4. Bactericides seem to cause an imbalance on the skin possibly leading to many skin disorders.

Chapter 13: Microbiology and Natural Products

Chemists argue that parabens are safe and that they protect people from microbiological growth in products. I believe they are correct when it comes to keeping bacteria, fungus and mold growth to a minimum to eliminating it. You already know my position about the potential harm of parabens destroying the natural probiotics of the skin. The reason I wrote this chapter is because eliminating parabens does not end the story, but actually begins a concern of mine for all natural products.

What is critical in this chapter is to learn how to use, store and buy natural products. Although many of us that make natural products use alternative to preserve our products, they are not as powerful and not as disruptive as parabens. Some of these ingredients include extracts like rosemary that slow microbiology growth in products and offer other features and benefits. Rosemary, for example, is also a natural antioxidant.

There are some critical facets to understand when buying and using natural products:

1. Freshness is one of the most important things to look for in natural products.

2. Rigorous testing of ingredients and finished goods.

3. Best used by dates that are reasonable, but not too long.

4. Permanent date and batch codes on the product packaging.

At Keys, we have a microbiology lab on site. All ingredients that come from raw material manufacturers and suppliers are tested to assure that the bacteria count is minimal and of the friendly kind. We test again after we have made the product and packaged it. Three samples of finished product are pulled at the front of the manufacturing run and at the end. We then use accelerated testing after a 72 hour incubation period looking for any bacteria growth and any unfriendly bacteria. Because we pretest the raw materials, we have not experienced a "run loss" where we have to destroy the batch. If we did see any gram-positive rods in a batch, we would destroy it.

Once a product has been tested to be safe, we etch using a laser both the "Best Used By Date" and batch code using a laser into either the bottle or the labels. This code cannot be altered

Why is this important?

All food and natural products that have not been irradiated or laced with parabens have bacteria. Like our skin, most things, especially earth derived products have both friendly and unfriendly bacteria.

Like our food, we choose to buy organic because it has no pesticides that are used during the growing process. Raw food is also free of any agents used to preserve them chemically. Some foods like apples are preserved by using simple inert gas that slows oxidation. Wine for example "sparges" nitrogen in the bottle prior to corking to remove air and slow oxidation. All of these example still have friendly bacteria present.

I often like to use the analogy of really fine quality blue cheese. My favorites are Rogue Blue and Maytag Blue. The blue part is injected bacteria that causes the cheese to basically mold. This taste treat is perfectly compatible with most people, but in truth, some people have allergies to cheese. This can be discrete where they are only allergic to soft cheeses and not hard cheeses. For some, they are allergic to all cheese. It is an important distinction because they are probably not reacting to the mold, but may be.

The same is true for our skin. Like our digestive track, the skin is also an organ that thrives on balance. The bacteria on our skin perform the function of supporting the skin as well as repelling bad bacteria, parasites and other forms of invaders.

For example, we find potentially harmful Staphylococcus on the skin as part of the normal condition. It is perfectly harmless when on the skin and coexists with other forms of bacteria. We get concerned when Staph invades an open wound where it is usually harmful.

So what is the point?

All natural substances have bacteria. Most of which is helpful and not harmful. These bacteria can morph or change over time and exposure to chemicals designed to destroy them. In natural cosmetics and personal care, it is obvious that we are dealing with different formulation methods and ingredients. This difference draws attention to the need to look at how we store, use and buy natural products.

Our customer service team averages about 25% of the questions that people submit to us asking, "when will Keys have large family sizes" of our products. This question is indicative of a society that has been conditioned to buying in bulk to save money and expense. The simple answer to this question is never!

The reason we do not make larger sizes deals with two facets. The first is freshness or efficacy and the second is a concern of how fast people use our products. Natural products that are water based have a much greater chance of oxidizing and forming mold after they are opened. This is also true of products that are near the pH of water. Alkaline soaps and products tend to be less bacterial friendly than mildly acidic products. Therefore, you will often see larger sizes of more alkaline soaps while the same manufacturer will only offer smaller sizes of lotions or cosmetics.

Packaging is also a big concern in regard to microbiology.

First, most manufacturers of bottles, jars and enclosures assume that the people filling them are using parabens. They therefore pay little concern to how the containers are shipped or boxed. Cardboard boxes not only harbor dirt, but microorganisms. If you do not clean these containers or request that they be separately individually wrapped, there is a strong likelihood that these containers already contain extra bacteria.

The good news is the industry is going green and clean which means that natural products makers can now buy containers especially designed to be cleaner and reduce oxidation.

For example, Keys was one of the first manufacturers to adopt airless containers over tubes. All of our full sized lotions are filled into a special package that keeps air and bacteria out of the container. Tubes can be easily contaminated once opened and by nature actually draw bacteria back inside. Next time you use a product packaged in a tube, when you push out the product, notice what happens to the small amount of product at the mouth of the tube. What you will notice is that a small amount of the product actually sucks back into the tube. Any bacteria that the product comes in contact with go back into the tube. This can further contaminate the entire tube.

Jars are the worst product container by far because not only is the jar open to the environment, we usually use our fingers to scoop out the product. Every time you rub or scoop product from an open jar, you are introducing bacteria into the product. Just leaving it open to the air exposes the entire surface to airborne bacteria.

At Keys, we only produce one product that uses a jar. Our Eye Butter is an eye cream that is mostly Shea butter and oils. Remember that I mentioned that bacteria like's water, so we do not use water in Eye Butter! The moisture comes from organic cucumber juice that is filtered and contained in such a way to minimize any bacteria growth. Said, part of the reason it is in a small 15ml (0.5 oz) jar is that we need you to use it quickly. Often for those people that live in a warm humid environment, I even recommend that they leave their Eye Butter in the refrigerator.

Bacteria are the enemy of natural products. Without preservatives like rosemary, it would be very tough to make viable products. Parabens would help, but are shown to harm our natural skin bacterial flora. In a perfect world, a targeted preservative would help us to make larger sizes. As technology progresses, there will be other solutions.

The biggest message here is that your use and buying habits need to change when it comes to natural cosmetics and skin care.

Chapter Tools

1. True natural products do not contain parabens.

2. Natural products use preservatives to retard bacteria growth.

3. Buy small containers more frequently for freshness and safety.

4. Avoid jars for softer thinner products opting for airless type containers.

5. When using jar products that contain water as an ingredient, use a disposable spatula to extract the product and then place on fingers.

6. Do not buy products in large containers that take over 6 months to use after opening.

Chapter 14: Organic Cosmetics and Skin Care

There are a couple of points I want to make about the use and abuse of the term 'organic'. Like the term 'natural', I have no desire to participate in a group session to define the term. So, I went to a friend that participates in the Organic Natural Skin Care business and asked him what definition he uses. He referred me to the Organic Trade Association. I went to their web site and extracted the following definition verbatim.

The National Organic Standards Board Definition of "Organic"

The following definition of "organic" was passed by the NOSB at its April 1995 meeting in Orlando, Florida.

"Organic agriculture is an ecological production management system that promotes and enhances biodiversity, biological cycles and soil biological activity. It is based on minimal use of off-farm inputs and on management practices that restore, maintain and enhance ecological harmony.

'Organic' is a labeling term that denotes products produced under the authority of the Organic Foods Production Act. The principal guidelines for organic production are to use materials and practices that enhance the ecological balance of natural systems and that integrate the parts of the farming system into an ecological whole.

Organic agriculture practices cannot ensure that products are completely free of residues; however, methods are used to minimize pollution from air, soil and water.

Organic food handlers, processors and retailers adhere to standards that maintain the integrity of organic agricultural products. The primary goal of organic agriculture is to optimize the health and productivity of interdependent communities of soil life, plants, animals and people."

I must admit that I read this and do not fully understand what it means. The reason I include it is to offer a reference to my two points.

Natural or organic is neither a feature or benefit!

So, I am standing in a Whole Foods Market in Portland Oregon. I am in the 'Whole Body' section of the store. I was early for a meeting in the Pearl District and decided to check out the latest and greatest products. At Keys we do not sell our products through Whole Foods for a raft of reasons, but I do know that they usually have the latest and greatest new natural products for cosmetic and body care.

What I first noticed was that there were all sorts of products offering different seals claiming to be organic. One product had four different seals on the back, front and side of the product. I had about a half hour before having to leave for the meeting, so I just kept reading labels. The more I read, the more something started to bug me. I could not put my finger on it and it was time to leave. Remember my nature is one of a curious scientist and it bothers me to no end to be perplexed by something. Especially something as simple as a logo on a label.

My meeting and demo was at Fez Studio. This is an eco chic skin apothecary in the historic Pearl District of Portland. I walked in the store and the owner chief designer was with a customer. He invited me over and introduced me as one of the founders of Keys. We began to chat about a problem this person visiting the store was having. We began to talk about the features, benefits and advantages of some skin care products and their being combined with some makeup. The customer was intense and had many questions. I thought to myself that I felt like I was on the tradeshow floor of a high tech computer convention. And it was at that point that it dawned on me what was perplexing me about the products with those organic seals affixed on them.

What dawned on me looking at all the personal care products while at Whole Foods is that the manufacturer consciously or unconsciously believes that organic and natural are a feature, benefit or advantage for their customers and over a competitor's product. Not!

After more than twenty years in high tech in Silicon Valley, a feature, benefit or advantage is something that directly benefits, has an advantage or is a feature that can be quantified. To me natural and organic fit more of a quality statement than features, benefits and advantages.

For example, I spent most of my high tech career in computer data storage. Take a hard disk as example of what I am talking about. When you buy a hard disk, if you are like most, you look for the highest capacity at the lowest price. If you are someone that plays computer games, your criteria is the fastest transfer rate, fastest access and then the disk with the greatest capacity. If you are an Information Technology (IT) person, you might be looking for capacity and compatibility. These are features, benefits and advantages. Bigger, faster cheaper!

Back to the Whole Foods shelves, I went after my meeting at Fez Studio. I grabbed the same products and looked at them for real features, benefits and advantages. To my delight, I actually found some that had them listed, but sad to say the majority did not. See, to me, real features and benefits are what a product does for you and what you can expect from it. If I use this organic shampoo, what will it do for me? Will my hair be cleaner, shinier, softer or stay cleaner longer? Does it rinse out faster? Will it help my scalp in some way? These are features and benefits.

Yes, truly organic products are safe as is natural because there is no junk. To me being natural and organic is a quality assurance and not feature or benefit. It is certainly not a competitive advantage because the shelves are full of the same claims.

A marketing professor once told me, "Products better make you feel good or solve a problem...Great products do both!" I guess you could say that natural and organic makes you feel good, but solving a problem by inferring that it is better does seem to push the envelope for me.

Look at the labels and ask yourself why am I considering this product? What will it do for me? How will I benefit from using it? What difference will it make in my life?

Well, if this confuses, then the next topic will surely make you wonder!

Organic Does Not Necessarily Mean Clean

Go back to the top of this chapter and read the definition of organic again. This time with the concept of what makes clean organic ingredients good enough to be safe to use them in cosmetic and personal care products.

A couple of years ago, I was invited to do a presentation on my perception of organic and clean products at a meeting of the Compact Signers for Safe Cosmetics. My speech title was" Organic does not Mean Green and Green does not mean Clean". In preparation for this meeting, I had befriended a scientist a year or so prior who headed up research for Max Zeller Phytopharmaceutical in Switzerland. We met at a conference and we spent a good amount of time talking about organics, clean processes and some new ways of thinking. Zeller is a herbal pharmaceutical company that grows all of its herbs in fields near their factory using very sophisticated sustainable processes. When I held my friend's company as an example, he quickly corrected me that Zeller was not the norm, but the exception. He continued that there are a few companies that are organic and have clean processes and that most organic labels really just mean grown without pesticides. I wondered is this another rewrite of "the king has no clothes."

I was so inspired by talking to him that I began to look at companies that were doing the same thing and found a few, but not a lot. He was right. Most everyone I talked to selling organic ingredients had a wide and varied definition.

I happened to be visiting Horst Rechelbacher, the founder of Aveda, now at his new operations in Minneapolis called Intelligent Nutrients. I shared the story about Max Zeller and he offered that he was doing the same thing on his herb farm in Wisconsin. This even inspired me more to seek out organic eco herbal farms to do something that I have been thinking of for a long time. Now I had two examples of companies doing what I needed, but sans becoming a farmer, the quest was not going well. I was getting a lot of fuel for my speech.

No to get too far off track, but I have had this idea of creating an herbal blend for the skin based on some probiotic principles. The same way as probiotics help the gut, I have an idea to do the same thing for the skin. So, all of this talk and discovery was a great incentive for me to explore my ideas.

Back on point, I started to look for organic herb farms around the country. What I discovered was unsettling and I wondered was it a trend, the norm or the exception. What I found was that although the herb farms did not use pesticides, most of their equipment included old rusty machines kept running with motor oil and various modifications. Yes, I found some very state-of-the-art facilities, but not in the US.

My project was put on hold for a number of reasons and I now had to prepare for my speech.

I gave my speech offering the following challenges in front of the green organic cosmetics and personal care manufacturers:

- Extracts, Botanicals & Herbal Solutions most likely contain parabens unless freeze-dried, dehydrated, frozen or refrigerated.

- Natural and organic do not mean the same thing to suppliers, manufacturers or end users.

- Ingredient grading and quality is declining with market growth.

- Green products have to be manufactured more like pharmaceuticals or high-grade food.

- Consumers need to be retrained and educated how green products differ from conventional.

- Organic does not mean green or clean!

- Some green products are not clean!

In short, here is what I discovered:

- There does not seem to be any over arching definition of organic that covers the origin and handling of ingredients with specific guidelines.

- Organic means without pesticides to most US farmers.

- Organic certification programs are questionable as to their authenticity.

- There are probably more organic labels than actual organic certifications.

Here are my parting thoughts. I look for products based on what they do to help me. I try to use as few as products as possible for simplicity sake. I buy natural almost exclusively for my foods and products. When possible, I buy organic.

I realize that this is a controversial subject and I wanted to include it in the book because I believe it is just another data point to consider when going natural and organic in your cosmetics and personal care.

Conclusions

You must certainly have noticed the close proximity that I hold between natural food, natural cosmetic and skin care products. This is because I believe they are all related. If you just hold in perspective my belief that what we put on our body is as important as what we put in it, you get this books meaning and purpose.

Maintaining skin balance is paramount. Understanding the effects and affects of chemicals in cosmetics and personal care products is paramount. Educating yourself to become a lifelong student of your own skin health will preserve your youth and your health.

The flora on our skin is like the atmosphere that surrounds the earth. It is life sustaining and vital. It protects and nourishes.

Further, chemicals in our cosmetics and personal care are recent inventions. The natural movement is not new, but more of a return to what was the norm 100 years ago.

I truly believe that many skin disorders are misdiagnosed and are actually caused by chemicals in the products we use. I am very concerned about the use of Triclosan and parabens in our cosmetics and personal care products. I am unnerved by their use in foods and dental care.

The good news is that I believe we are seeing the beginning of a trend to a lifestyle that is more natural and conservative. Said, we have a long way to go. What we have concocted as a chemicals society has taken us nearly 100 years to construct. It may only take half that time to get back to the future.

Again, if there is only one thing that you take away from this book, it is "What you put on your body is as important as what you put in it."

✚ Resources

The **Campaign for Safe Cosmetics** has the **Skin Deep** database where you can search for safe personal care and cosmetics products

www.safecosmetics.org

TOXNET - Databases on toxicology, hazardous chemicals, environmental health, and toxic releases is maintained by the United States National Institutes of Health and the National Medical Library

http://toxnet.nlm.nih.gov/

Clean Green Cafe is a blog and chat forum sponsored by Keys and is focused on education. It is the extension of this book.

www.CleanGreenCafe.com

Teens Turning Green is an offshoot of The Search for the Cause organization that was the Marin County Cancer Project. This is a great resource for young adults and teens.

www.TeensTurningGreen.com

There are many resources and these are among the best. You can stay tuned on Clean Green Cafe for additional resources

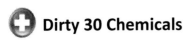 Dirty 30 Chemicals

The Dirty Thirty. A Reprised Dirty Dozen... 30 Bad Boy Chemicals!

A number of years ago, a few concerned people in Marin County California wondered why cancer rates were so high in their community. With the support of George Lucas and at the hand of Judy Shils, the Marin County Cancer Project was born. One of the first things that they realized was that there were certain chemicals used in personal care products. They identified them as contributing to elevated cancer rates and tagged them with the name, "The Dirty Dozen." Many of these chemicals are now known to be harmful and the research a direct response to the efforts of the Marin County Cancer Project.

Now known as the "Search For the Cause", the project realized that they must influence the younger members of our community and created another organization called "Teens Turning Green". This group has now carried on the tradition and has expanded the list to thirty.

We are pleased to present the Dirty Thirty as chemicals of grave concern in everyday personal care and household products.

Note: Keys scientists have reviewed this list and have noted research papers on each chemical showing evidence of the claims below. We note that it is the burden of the manufacturers of human and pet products that use these chemicals to prove to a point of certainty to their customers that these chemicals are safe. We support continued research and testing on all ingredients whether they are synthetic, organic or natural for safety and toxicity. Keys does not use any of the Dirty Thirty Chemicals based on questionable danger to humans and animals.

DIRTY THIRTY

1. **CHEMICAL: ALUMINUM ZIRCONIUM and OTHER ALUMINUM COMPOUNDS**

Function: Used to control sweat and odor in the underarms by slowing down the production of sweat

Present in: Antiperspirants. Banned by EU.

Health concerns: Linked to the development of Alzheimer's Disease; may be linked to breast cancer; probable neurotoxin; possible nervous system, respiratory, and developmental toxin.

2. **CHEMICAL: BENZYL ACETATE**

Function: Solvent; hidden within "fragrance."

Present in: Many cosmetics and personal care products, read labels.

Health concerns: Linked to pancreatic cancer; easily absorbs into skin causing quick systemic effects; animal studies show hyperemia of the lungs; possible gastrointestinal, liver, and respiratory toxicant; possible neurotoxin.

3. **CHEMICAL: BENZALKONIUM CHLORIDE and BENZETHONIUM CHLORIDE**

Function: Antimicrobial agent, deodorant, preservative, biocide.

Present in: Moisturizer, sunscreen, facial cleanser, acne treatment, pain relief. Restricted in Japan and Canada.

Health concerns: Immune system toxicant; may trigger asthma; possible organ system toxicant; animal studies show endocrine disruption and brain, nervous system, respiratory and blood effects; possible carcinogen.

4. CHEMICAL: BRONOPOL

Function: Preservative.

Present in: Moisturizer, body wash, facial cleanser, makeup remover, anti-aging products. Restricted in Canada.

Health concerns: Immune system toxicant; lung and skin toxicant; animal studies show endocrine disruption and gastrointestinal, brain and nervous system effects; irritant.

5. CHEMICAL: BUTYL ACETATE

Function: Solvent in polishes and treatments, prevents chipping.

Present in: Nail polish and nail treatments.

Health concerns: Repeated exposure causes skin dryness and cracking; vapors may induce drowsiness or dizziness; flammable.

6. CHEMICAL: BUTYLATED HYDROXYTOLUENE (BHT)/ BUTYLATED HYDROXYANISOLE (BHA)

Function: Anti-Oxidant; slows down the rate at which product ingredients change in color.

Present in: Many cosmetics and personal care products, read labels.

Banned by EU.

Health Concerns: Immune system toxicant; endocrine disruptor; probable human carcinogen; animal studies show brain, liver, neurotoxin, reproductive and respiratory toxicant.

7. CHEMICAL: ETHOXYLATED INGREDIENTS:CETEARETH/PEG COMPOUNDS

Function: Surfactant, emulsifying or cleansing agent, penetration enhancer.

Present in: Many cosmetics and personal care products, read labels.

Health concerns: Animal studies show brain, nervous system and sense organ effects; irritant; reproductive and skin toxin, alters skin structure, allowing other chemicals to penetrate deep into the skin and increasing the amounts of other chemicals that reach the bloodstream; may contain harmful impurities.

8. CHEMICAL: COAL TAR

Function: Controls itching and eczema, softens and promotes the dissolution of hard, scaly, rough skin, also used in hair dyes.

Present in: Shampoo and Hair Dye. Banned by Canada and EU.

Health concerns: Known human carcinogen; skin and respiratory toxicant.

9. CHEMICAL: COCAMIDE DEA/ LAURAMIDE DEA

Function: used as foaming agents in shampoos and bath products, and as emulsifying agents in cosmetics; foaming and cleansing agents for "mouth feel."

Present in: Many cosmetics and personal care products, read labels.

Health concerns: Human immune system toxicant; forms carcinogenic nitrosamine compounds if mixed with nitrosating agents; animal studies show sense organ effects and skin irritation; may contain harmful impurities.

10. CHEMICAL: DIETHANOLAMINE (DEA)

Function: pH adjuster.

Present in: Sunscreen, moisturizer, foundation, hair color.

Health concerns: Skin and immune system toxicant; possible carcinogen; irritant; animal studies show endocrine disruption and neuro developmental, brain and nervous system effects; may trigger asthma.

11. CHEMICAL: ETHYL ACETATE

Function: Solvent.

Present in: Nail polish products, mascara, tooth whitening, perfume.

Health concerns: Probable neurotoxin; possible nervous system toxin; possible carcinogen; irritant; highly flammable

12. CHEMICAL: FORMALDEHYDE

Function: Disinfectant, germicide, fungicide, preservative.

Present in: Deodorant, nail polish, soap, shampoo, shaving cream. Restricted in Canada. Banned by EU.

Health concerns: Immune system, repertory, hematological, and skin toxicant; probable carcinogen and cardiovascular toxicant; can damage DNA; may trigger asthma; animal studies show sense organ, brain, and nervous system effects; possible human development toxicant.

13. CHEMICAL: FORMALDEHYDE-RELEASING PRESERVATIVES (QUATERNIUM-15, DMDM HYDANTOIN, DIAZOLIDINYL UREA AND IMIDAZOLIDINYL UREA, DEA, MEA, TEA)

Function: Anti-microbial preservative.

Present in: Many cosmetics and personal care products, read labels.

Health concerns: Forms nitrosamines when in the presence of amines such as MEA, DEA and TEA; probable immune system, blood, cardiovascular and skin toxicant; possible carcinogen; animal studies show endocrine disruption, nervous system and organ system effects; may contain harmful impurities.

14. CHEMICAL: FRAGRANCE (PARFUM)

Function: Deodorant, masking, perfuming

Present in: Many cosmetics and personal care products, read labels.

Health concerns: Immune system toxicant; possible neurotoxin; can contain between 10 and 300 different chemicals, many of which have never been tested for safety; see phthalates. Labeling can be confusing. If uncertain, check with manufacturer.

15. CHEMICAL: HYDROQUINONE

Function: Antioxidant, fragrance ingredient, skin bleaching agent, hair colorant.

Present in: Skin fading/lightener, facial moisturizer, anti-aging, sunscreen, hair color, facial cleanser and moisturizer. Restricted in Canada.

Health concerns: Immune system and respiratory toxicant; probable neurotoxin; possible carcinogen; irritant; animal studies show endocrine disruption.

16. CHEMICAL: IODOPROPYNYL BUTYLCARBAMATE

Function: Preservative.

Present in: Many cosmetics and personal care products, read labels. Restricted in Japan.

Health concerns: Human toxicant; possible liver immune system toxin; allergenic.

17. CHEMICAL: LEAD and LEAD COMPOUNDS

Function: Colorant.

Present in: Hair dye, hair products. Traces found in some red lipstick. Restricted in Canada.

Health concerns: Probable carcinogen; developmental, respiratory, gastrointestinal and reproductive toxicant; reduced fertility; animal studies show metabolic, brain and nervous system effects; suspected nano-scale ingredients with potential to absorb into the skin.

18. CHEMICAL: METHYLISOTHIAZOLINONE (MI/MCI) and METHYLCHLOROISOTHAIZOLINONE

Function: Preservative.

Present in: Many cosmetics and personal care products, read labels. Restricted in Canada and Japan.

Health concerns: Immune system toxicant; animal studies show restricted growth of the axons and dendrites of immature nerves, neurotoxicity and positive mutation results; can lead to a malfunction in the way neurons communicate with each other; especially detrimental to a developing nervous system.

19. CHEMICAL: Oxybenzone (BENZPENONE-3)

Function: Sunscreen Agent; Ultraviolet Light Absorber, UV Absorber; UV Filter.

Present in: Sunscreens and makeup

Health concerns: Associated with photoallergic reactions and immunotoxicity. Probable carcinogen and endocrine disrupter; Enhanced skin absorption and bioaccumulates to dangerous levels; biochemical cellular changes. Developmental and reproductive toxicity.

20. CHEMICAL: PARABENS (METHYL, ETHYL, PROPYL AND BUTYL)

Function: Preservative and anti-bacterial agent.

Present in: Many cosmetics and personal care products, read labels.

Health concerns: May alter hormone levels, possibly increasing risk for certain types of cancer, impaired fertility, or alteration of the development of a fetus or young child; studies have found parabens in breast tumors; probable skin toxicant; animal studies show brain and nervous system effects.

21. CHEMICAL: PETROLATUM (PETROLEUM)

Function: Forms barrier on skin; makes lipsticks shine and creams smoother; inexpensive skin softener.

Present in: Many cosmetics and personal care products, read labels. Banned by EU.

Health concerns: May be contaminated with impurities, linked to cancer or other significant health problems.

22. CHEMICAL: PHTHALATES (DIBUTYL PHTHALATES)

Function: Fragrance ingredient, plasticizer, solvent.

Present in: Many cosmetics and personal care products, read labels. Banned in EU.

Health concerns: Immune system toxicant; developmental and reproductive toxin; respiratory toxicant; probable neurotoxin; possible carcinogen and endocrine disruptor; bio-accumulative in wildlife.

23. CHEMICAL: P-PHENYLENEDIAMINE (PPD)

Function: Hair colorant.

Present in: Hair dye, shampoo, hair spray. Restricted in Canada.

Health concerns: Immune system and respiratory toxicant; probable neurotoxin; eczema; possible nervous system, skin, kidney and liver toxicant; irritant; may trigger asthma and gastritis; shown to cause cancer in animal studies.

24. CHEMICAL: PROPYLENE GLYCOL

Function: Solvent, penetration enhancer, conditions skin, controls viscosity and keeps products from melting in high temperatures or freezing when it is cold.

Present in: Many cosmetics and personal care products, read labels.

Health concerns: Alters skin structure, allowing other chemicals to penetrate deep into the skin and increasing the amounts of other chemicals that reach the bloodstream; animal studies show reproductive effects, positive mutation results, brain and nervous system effects and endocrine disruption.

25. CHEMICAL: SODIUM LAURETH SULFATE

Function: Surfactant, penetration enhancer.

Present in: Many cosmetics and personal care products, read labels.

Health concerns: Alters skin structure, allowing other chemicals to penetrate deep into the skin, increasing the amounts of other chemicals that reach the bloodstream; Irritant; animal studies show sense organ effects.

26. CHEMICAL: TALC

Function: Absorbs moisture, anti-caking agent, bulking agent.

Present in: Blush, powder, eye shadow, baby powder, deodorant.

Health concerns: Carcinogen; link between talcum powder and ovarian cancer; talc particles are similar to asbestos particles and data suggests that it can cause tumors in the lungs; probable respiratory toxin.

27. CHEMICAL: TOLUENE

Function: Antioxidant, solvent to improve adhesion and gloss.

Present in: Nail polish and hair dye.

Health concerns: Liver toxin; probable developmental, nervous system and respiratory toxin; possible cardiovascular, musculoskeletal, renal and sense organ toxin; possible carcinogen and reproductive toxin; irritant; highly flammable.

28. CHEMICAL: TRICLOSAN

Function: Anti-bacterial agent, deodorant, preservative, biocide. Reduces and controls bacterial contamination on the hands and on treated products.

Present in: Antibacterial soaps, deodorants, toothpastes, mouthwashes, face wash and cleaning supplies. Restricted in Japan and Canada.

Health concerns: Probable endocrine disrupter and carcinogen; easily bio-accumulates to dangerous levels; irritant; animal studies show reproductive and other broad systematic effects; potentially contaminated with impurities linked to cancer and other significant health problems; studies have shown it can actually induce cell death when used in mouth washes.

29. CHEMICAL: TREITHANOLAMINE (TEA)

Function: Fragrance ingredient, pH adjuster, surfactant.

Present in: Hand & body lotion, shaving creams, soap, shampoo, bath powders and moisturizer.

Health concerns: Immune system toxicant; possible carcinogen; animal studies show endocrine disruption; may trigger asthma; forms carcinogenic nitrosamine compounds if mixed with nitrosating agents.

30. CHEMICAL: 1,4 DIOXANE

Function: Penetration enhancer

Present in: Body lotion, moisturizers, sunless tanning products, baby soap, anti-aging products..

Health concerns: EPA classifies it as a probable carcinogen found in 46 of 100 personal care products marketed as organic or natural, and the National Toxicology Program considers it a known animal carcinogen. Acute (short-term) inhalation exposure to high levels of 1,4 dioxane has caused vertigo, drowsiness, headache, anorexia and irritation of the eyes, nose, throat and lungs of humans. It may also irritate the skin.